"I had knee problems starting in my twenties. Since I love to move my body, this meant countless hours in the gym and many visits to physical therapists over the years. All this helped somewhat, but it was only after discovering Balance techniques that everything fell into place. At that point I had not run for two years due to increasing difficulties, and I was worried that my knee problems would affect other pursuits such as swimming and biking. Within days of being introduced to Balance, I ran my first kilometer. Now, more than 18 months later, I still run regularly with virtually no difficulty. Balance made an enormous difference. I would have a hard time believing this, had it not happened to me. Pinch me—I am a very happy athlete!"

~ *Per-Magnus Skoogh, Managing Director, mPeira, Göteborg, Sweden*

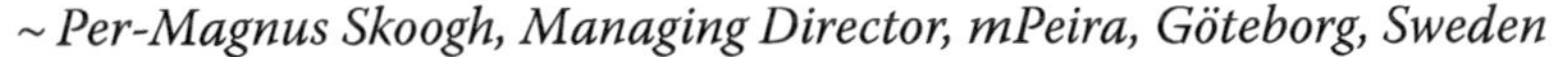

"As a sleep specialist, my experience with this training has given me an increased awareness of alignment and how the body balances around the spine. Balance is sound advice. Integrating these simple yet profound techniques into the bedtime ritual holds great promise for improving sleep quality and will maximize the health benefits that come from sound restful sleep, without pain."

~ *Sharon Keenan, Ph.D., Director, The School of Sleep Medicine, Inc., Palo Alto, CA*

"As a massage therapist specializing in orthopedic conditions, I find Balance/Aplomb to be a crucial component of my work. Clients experience lasting improvement and do not come back with the same aches and chronic tension. Without Balance, this would not occur. I benefit as well: I am able to sustain my strenuous workload and client volume. And as an avid dancer of Argentine tango, I can't praise enough how my dancing has improved with Balance!"

~ *Monika Hartwig, Therapeutic Massage Therapist, Palo Alto, CA*

"Two years ago I went to a standing-room-only concert at The Fillmore in San Francisco. I had back pain for most of the evening. Two weeks ago I went to a concert at the same place and, after standing for over two hours, I had no back pain. What a fabulous improvement! I could hardly believe it!"

~ *Fran Fisher, CPA, San Jose, CA*

"As a physical therapist and chiropractor I can highly recommend these teachings. This approach frees the body to function according to its original design. Once the principles are understood and mastered, pain and discomfort can be greatly relieved or eliminated."

~ *Petra Eggert, D.C., P.T., Cupertino, CA*

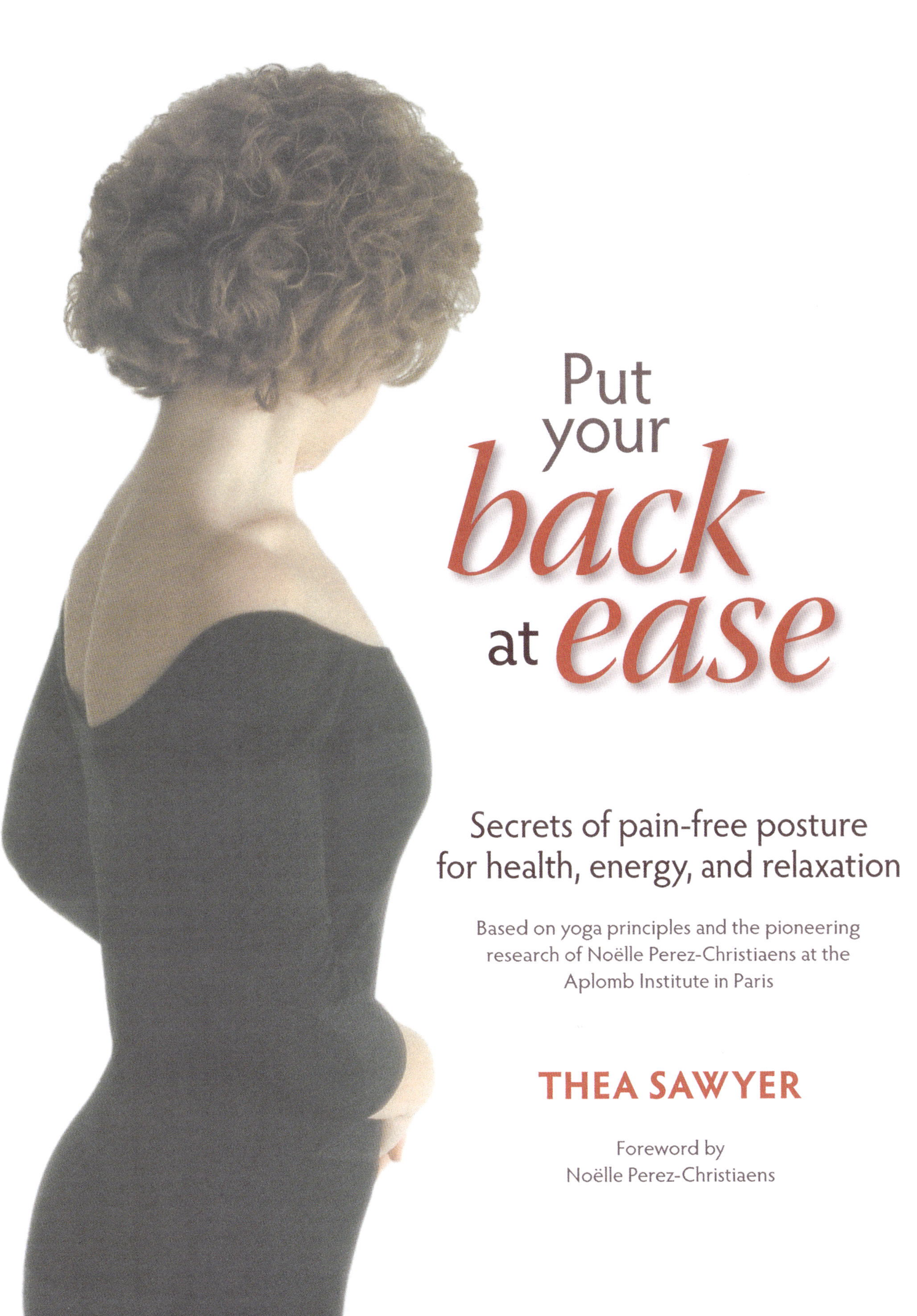

Put your *back* at *ease*

Secrets of pain-free posture for health, energy, and relaxation

Based on yoga principles and the pioneering research of Noëlle Perez-Christiaens at the Aplomb Institute in Paris

THEA SAWYER

Foreword by
Noëlle Perez-Christiaens

Put Your Back at Ease:
Secrets of pain-free posture for health, energy, and relaxation

Consult your physician before you begin this program. Do not push yourself beyond what your physical condition can support. The author and publisher are not responsible for any injury that might result from this practice.

ISBN-13: 978-0615856360

Editing by Darlene Frank
Book design and layout by Patricia Koren, Kajun Design
Front cover design by Sukha Carfagno
Front cover photographs by Robert Weaver (left) and Pier Luigi De Masi (right)
Studio photographs by Robert Weaver and Michael DiGiacomo

For quantity discounts, please contact Thea Sawyer at thea@liveinbalance.com.

This book is dedicated to
Nöelle Perez-Christiaens, who had the insight
to question, observe, and discover why
so many people suffer from back and joint pain,
and how to reverse the trend. Nöelle's work
is the foundation of this book.

ACKNOWLEDGMENTS

Deepest thanks to my teacher Nöelle Perez-Christiaens, who changed my life and the lives of many who were living in pain. While studying with her at the Aplomb Institute (ISA)[1] in Paris, I was blessed with the additional insights of senior teachers Georgia Leconte and Ginette Guedu. Each revealed a different view of the path toward realignment and healing. Miguel Fonseca, Nöelle's husband, was ever present to show us how to be at ease and feel light—thank you, Miguel, for your patience and willingness to let us observe you endlessly!

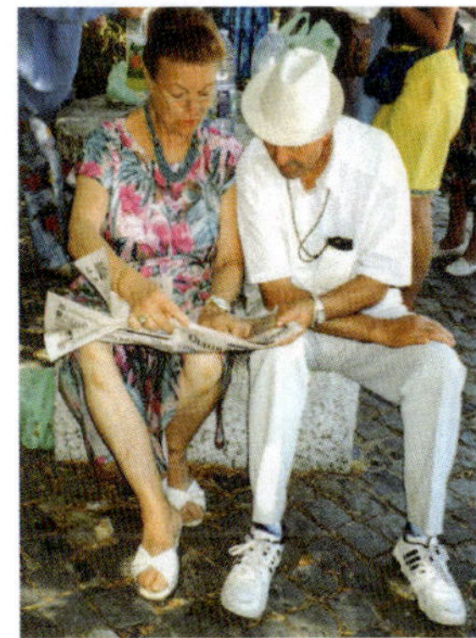

Nöelle and Miguel in Portugal.

This book represents the wishes of many to help promote the work of Nöelle Perez-Christiaens as it becomes more widely known in the U.S. under a variety of names. Since 1992 Jean Couch and her students at the Balance Center in Palo Alto, California have refined their understanding of this work, which continues to evolve. Much of the terminology developed at the Balance Center is used in this book. Jean's unflagging enthusiasm inspires all of us who teach and study there, and we continue to learn together.

I extend special thanks to the following people who have generously contributed to this book. In Darlene Frank I discovered the blessings of a superb editor. I am deeply grateful for her vital support in transforming the manuscript into this book. Sukha Carfagno modeled the poses and designed the book cover. Janet Buce Cook reviewed early drafts and provided insightful feedback. Jean Couch and the Balance Center provided a photographer and studio for the practice poses. Joanne Ehrich and Sukha Carfagno inspired the book's title.

I also thank the many subjects whose photographs are used to illustrate Balance. Where these photographs are not my own, they were generously contributed by Jean Couch and Janet Buce Cook, along with Georgia Leconte and Nöelle Perez-Christiaens. Other photo and illustration sources include Dreamstime.com, the Library of Congress, and the Smithsonian Institution. The illustration on page 14 is by Lidwine Houben Design, Nijmegen, The Netherlands.

Finally, I would like to express my love and gratitude to my husband, Tom. His steady support over the years made it possible for me to study in Paris and, in turn, to write this book.

CONTENTS

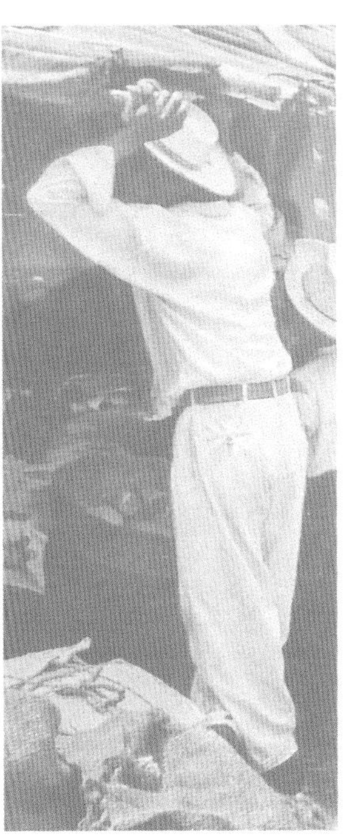

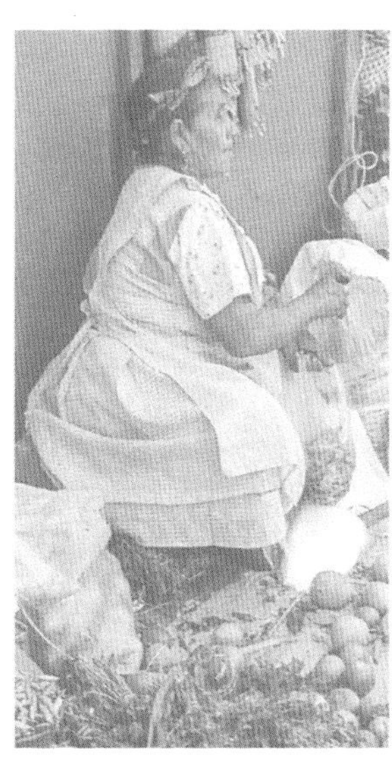

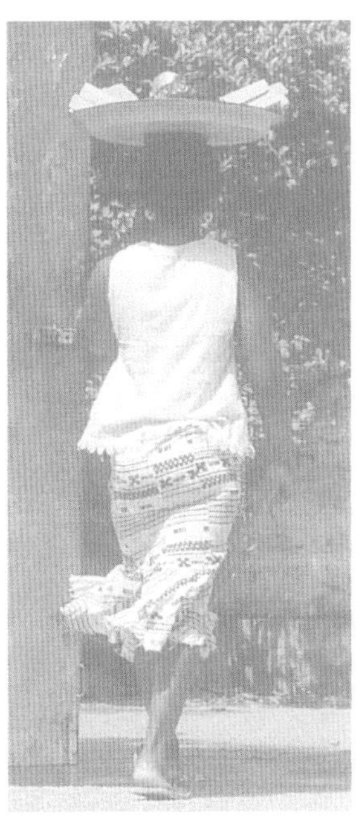

FOREWORD

By Nöelle Perez-Christiaens

"Put your back at ease." What does this mean? Do we mean the physical ease and upright bearing of our great-grandparents, passed down from generation to generation over thousands of years? Or is it the "ease" that our culture has adopted over the last century or so, of slouching or holding ourselves artificially? Is it the upright, loose-limbed posture that still exists among nine-tenths of the world's population, or this new way of leaning and slumping that many consider the norm for comfort and ease?

For many years I practiced a very strict yoga according to what I thought were the demands of my teacher, B. K. S. Iyengar. But by 1982, after 23 years of study, I was crippled with pain. Why? After much searching I ended up in Portugal. For various reasons I decided to settle in the city of Setubal to study the longshoremen there, who carried heavy loads on their heads all day long and for many years. How did they preserve such stately bearing? They did not appear to have back or neck pain. I thought they might help me understand how to achieve the yoga poses that hurt me. And this is how my husband, Miguel, and his family and co-workers, plus many other Portuguese, came into my life.

Let's return to our question: What does it mean to be at ease? Family photo albums often reveal our grandmothers sitting very upright yet looking beautiful, elegant, and relaxed. How did they do it? How did our grandfathers manage to maintain such firm, high buttocks into old age? How did they manage to stand with so much weight in their heels, their pelvis so far back that the points of their shoes lifted slightly?

How do Miguel, his sisters, and many others sit so upright and relaxed, the spine's natural arch well formed, chest wide and high, without leaning against the back of a chair? How do they sit so beautifully straight?

Comparing past and present reveals some interesting contrasts. For instance, I observed that our grandparents were straight like the letter **I**, whereas we are stooped and suffer from back pain. I have known elderly people who were practically bent in two from a serious injury, but the great majority remained straight until their death, with the natural arch of the spine still distinctly shaped.

Today it seems that humans have no shape: Pants and skirts hang badly; buttocks are flabby and droop pear-like. In the past, buttocks had the shape of an apple: round and firm. Men and women now have a rounded back. Looking at Miguel, his friends, and others in profile, you can draw a vertical line from the middle of their heads to their heels and that line will pass through the trochanters and a well-defined natural arch of the spine. The miracle is that these people seem to maintain a consistent level of physical relaxation. They work hard but use only the necessary muscles, while all the others are relaxed. The active muscles relax as soon as their action is finished.

I see this clearly on Miguel as he walks, adjusts a heavy weight he is carrying, or stands at the counter to scale the fish for dinner.

In contrast, the people I see on the street or in our classes at the Aplomb Institute have tense muscles. They strain, unaware, to maintain an artificial balance. From heels to pubic bone their vertical line swerves forward, then from pubic bone to the middle of the thoracic spine it moves back, then forward again along the upper spine and neck. The head is positioned with the nose up in the air. They have a zigzag shape. Imagine the brain in this artificial position—how can it float in its cerebrospinal fluid in its natural, horizontal position?

Fashion contributes to these distortions. It wants us to flatten the natural arch as we sit. The weight of the pelvis then falls back; in counterweight the thorax falls forward, the chin rises and the skull hangs back, creasing the neck. The chest is unnaturally lifted, causing the back to arch in the middle of the thoracic spine. All this is inflicted on the spine because of a posture that did not appear in France until after the First World War and that became more ingrained as lifestyles changed and fashions followed.

Should we stay in this new, so-called equilibrium that is destroying our bodies and causing pain? If not, how can we regain the balance that evolved naturally over thousands of years?

The secret is in the position of the pelvis. When you stand, you must before all else move the pelvis—the base of the spine—farther back toward the line of balance. Position your pelvis as if you were getting ready to sit down, which places your weight into your heels. You have to accept this feeling of being slightly seated when standing or walking. For many people in the world, this is natural. From this foundation the spine can regain its equilibrium and the breath can resume the mechanics of filling the whole chest space. The diaphragm never drops down; to the contrary, it rises and enlarges gently, all by itself. It does not press down against the digestive organs. It works gently, softly, joyously, and without intervention—because it is natural!

I have observed this pattern of the breath in people around the world in over 40 years of research.

On the axis of gravity everything on earth stays upright without effort. To align yourself with that axis will take time and attention. Didn't Mr. Iyengar ask his students to have "an attention that watches over the attention so that it does not escape"? Little by little, alignment will become easier and our day-to-day activities will tire us so much less. Out of alignment we need to use extra effort to hold ourselves upright. As a result we live in perpetual tension without being aware of it, and it tires us enormously. When we recover the natural balance of the human body we save energy, preserve our health, and find a profound joy in daily life.

It's not easy, but it is critical in order to become a "normal" human being again! This is what Miguel taught me.

By trying to copy Miguel's posture, I recovered my health and finally understood the profound, yet simple foundation of B. K. S. Iyengar's teachings. I urge you to learn this way for yourself. You will discover how good it feels to stand, sit, and move in this natural way, and you will become so much more beautiful.

Miguel and I hope that you will persevere in this search, following the example of our dear Thea.

Paris, France
November 2012

Translated by Thea Sawyer

A YOGA TEACHER'S QUEST

Put Your Back at Ease is about feeling healthy: energetic, pain-free, and joyful. It is based on the revolutionary insights of Nöelle Perez-Christiaens, who has been in tireless pursuit of physical ease and lightness since 1959, having experienced a taste of it as a yoga teacher studying in India with yoga master B. K. S. Iyengar. Moments of exquisite lightness made her believe that ease was possible, yet pain kept her from achieving it consistently in yoga or in daily life. What was missing?

The question lingered even after she left India. Mr. Iyengar had instructed her to walk behind the women of India and observe and copy them: "When your shadow matches theirs you will have made progress."[2] She could not do it. But the challenge set her on a path of travel and inquiry to observe and learn from cultures where people walked like the Indian women, gracefully upright and strong.

Nöelle began her research in Burkina Faso, Africa, continued her quest in Europe on the island of Madeira, and finally found in Portugal what she was looking for.

There, in the port of Setubal, she asked a group of *descargadeiros* (longshoremen) if she could study them, including analyzing X-rays of their spines. The workers' job was to offload fishing boats, carrying heavy platters of fish on their heads, walking a narrow gangplank from the boat and then to the nearby *lota* where the fish were sold. She was impressed by the energy, strength, and youthful bearing of these men, who seemed to be physically at ease in everything they did.

One of them, Miguel Fonseca, became her husband and primary teacher. Although it was difficult for him to describe the daily activities he did naturally and had never analyzed, she kept asking questions. Over time the two of them traveled in Portugal, Turkey, Morocco, Egypt, Mexico, Guatemala, Indonesia, and many other countries to study people who moved with the same grace and ease as the longshoremen. All these people became Nöelle's teachers. She not only observed how they looked but also how they lived, by lodging in simple accommodations like theirs and sharing their way of life.

Teaching others what she learned became her life's work. Her empirical research and studies of ethnophysiology[3] led to original conclusions that are steadily gaining recognition in the U.S. Nöelle has been a pioneer in blending the elements of natural posture with the holistic mind-body spirit of yoga. She insists that the physical body does not exist independently from its mental and spiritual aspects, and that real change is possible only when the whole person is involved.

This book is an invitation to experience yourself in a way that feels new, yet that you may vaguely remember from when you were a child. Its aim is to help you discover effortlessness in all you do—sitting at the computer, washing dishes, walking, playing the piano, and more.

You will discover the lightness that comes when your bones bear weight, releasing muscle tension and allowing greater freedom of movement. Such relaxation invites the attention and awareness you would bring to yoga, so that the postures of everyday life become *asanas* (yoga poses).

You will discover habitual tensions that you have not been aware of. And you will learn "not by memorizing postures and directions, but by discovering the law of balance, the mysteries of the human skeleton, the trap of tension, and the capacity to go always further into relaxation." [4]

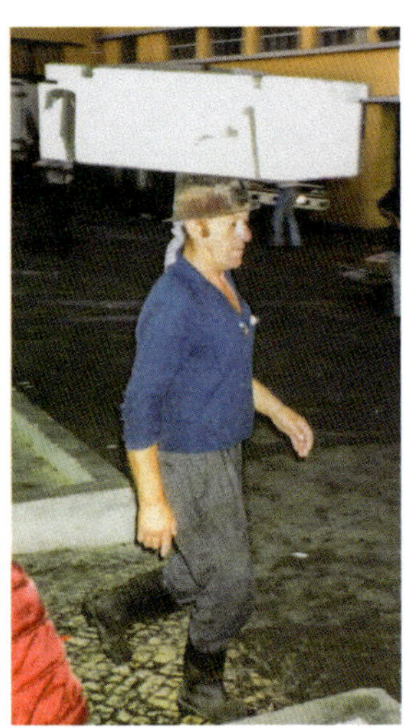

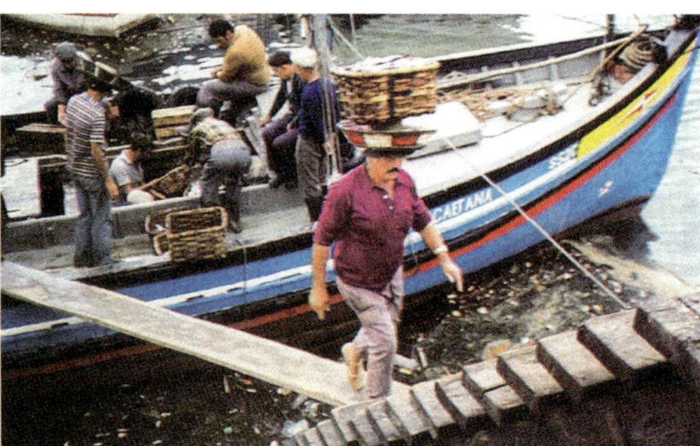

Portuguese descargadeiros *offloading fish from boat to auction.*

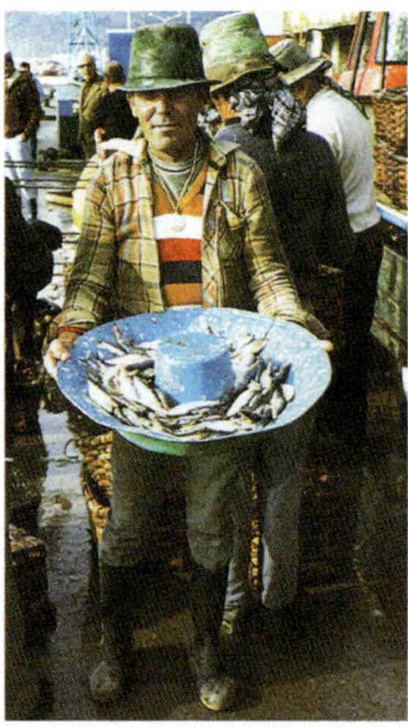

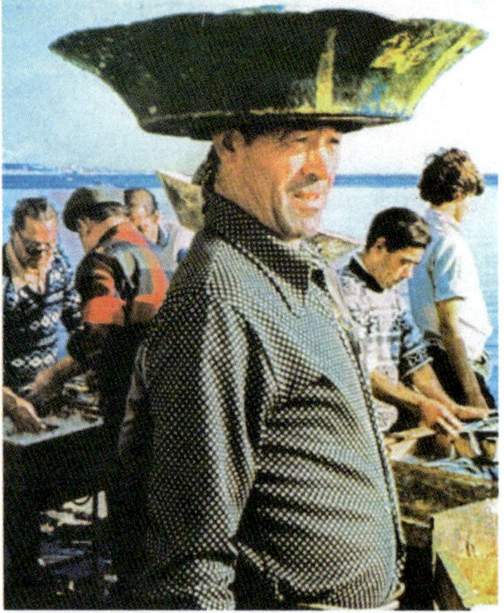

Miguel Fonseca.

HOW TO USE THIS BOOK

Anyone who has ever practiced yoga or tried to excel at a sport knows there is no substitute for one-on-one instruction with a good teacher or coach. Even professional athletes at the top of their form have coaches.

Although the techniques in this book will increase awareness of your current movement patterns, a book cannot teach you the finer points of how to change them. Hands-on instruction is essential to fully benefit and discover how to be relaxed and aligned. You will not need to learn new mechanical skills; rather you will unlearn habits that cause injury and strain. The physical ease you experience as you incorporate these new movement patterns into your life will keep you energetic, upright, and graceful.

This book, then, is intended to complement and reinforce what you learn with a teacher.

A word of caution: Do not use the information in this book as a substitute for medical treatment. If you have musculoskeletal pain, consult your physician before you begin using these techniques. Do not push yourself beyond what your physical condition can support.

Part 1 of this book introduces the foundations for discovering ease and what in this book is called "Balance," and the research on which these teachings are based. It describes what Balance looks and feels like, and which parts of the body play the most critical roles in achieving pain-free posture.

Part 2 provides specific practice guidelines for sitting, standing, bending, walking, and lying down in ways that will both relieve and prevent pain. This book reveals little-known but revolutionary insights to bring you pain relief, health, and vitality.

These findings have changed the lives of many people. They can change yours, too! Welcome to the world of ease and relaxation.

Part 1

FOUNDATIONS OF BALANCE AND EASE

We must sense to know.

~ Genevieve Brady[5]

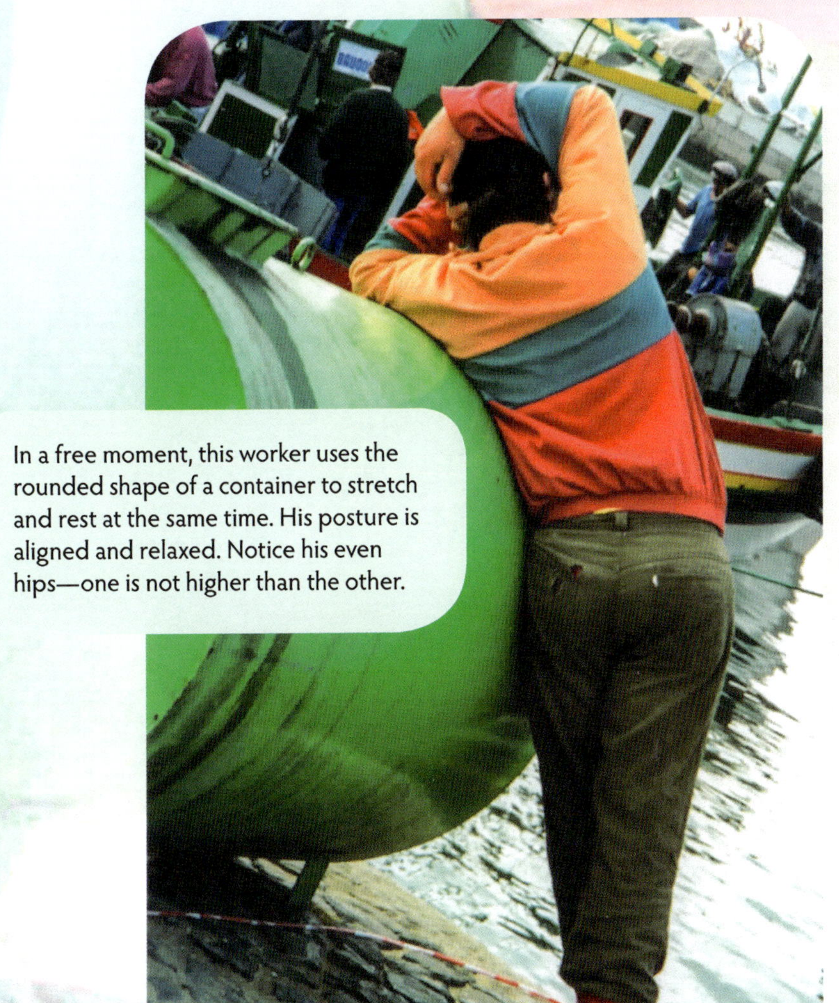

In a free moment, this worker uses the rounded shape of a container to stretch and rest at the same time. His posture is aligned and relaxed. Notice his even hips—one is not higher than the other.

FINDING THE KEY

The balancing power of the Zuni maiden is so perfect that she can carry a heavy water jug, poised upon her head, and run up the hundreds of rough-hewn steps to her lofty pueblo home.

~ Maud Smith Williams[6]

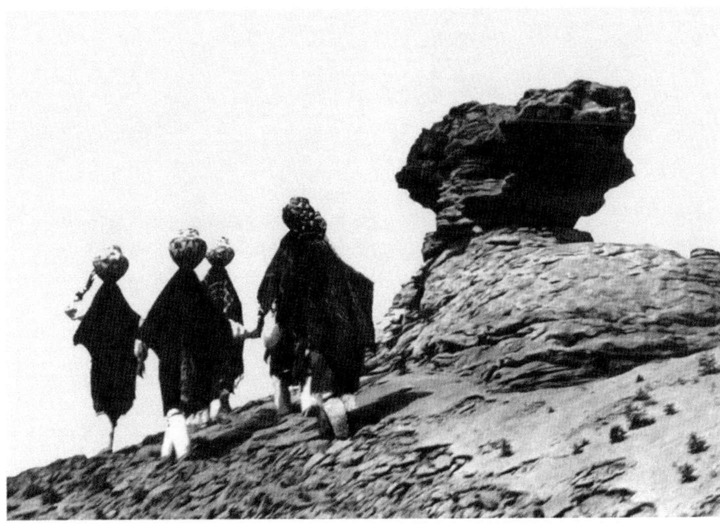

Acoma Water Girls, *by Edward S. Curtis, 1904.*

Imagine walking or running for extended periods of time or up a long flight of stairs and feeling energized rather than tired. Visualize being able to bend, stoop, lift, and carry with ease and without pain, to move gracefully and sleep deeply.

Sustaining intense activity at length comes naturally to the Rarámuri Indians of Mexico (also known as the Tarahumara, famous for being fast runners) and to many people in other parts of the world whose livelihood depends on their physical well-being. These people live primarily in rural areas. They do not suffer the back and joint pain so common in the U.S. They look graceful, strong, and energetic, and remain productive into old age. What is their secret?

Why does a Portuguese salt carrier in his fifties who carries 70 pounds of salt on his head many times a day not complain of back pain, while his son's back aches? Why do we see people "from the old country" in better shape than their children who are stooped and complain of fatigue? Why do Western yoga students get injured practicing an art of well-being that has endured for thousands of years?

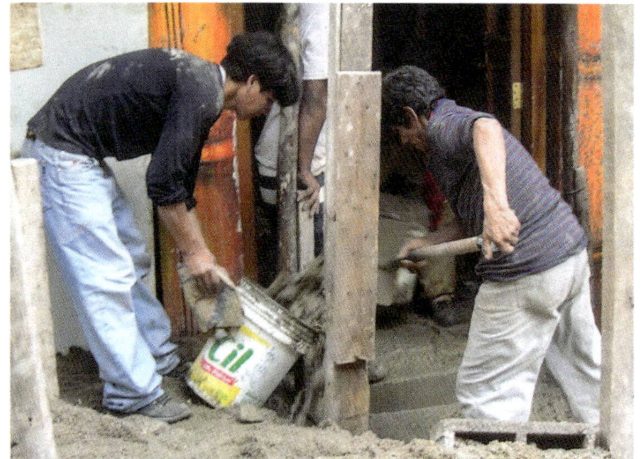

The older Peruvian man at right maintains a long spine while working. The younger man rounds his back and locks his knees and hips. Who looks more likely to get tired or injured?

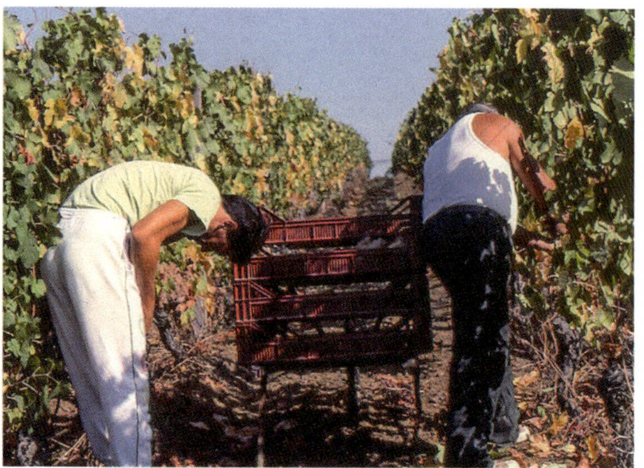

A father and son harvest grapes in Italy. Note the difference in their backs. Who looks weaker?

Questions like these captivated Nöelle Perez-Christiaens as she set out to find the key to lightness and ease. Initially her questions were triggered by her difficulty with Sirsasana, the headstand. She had practiced this pose for many years, following Iyengar's precise instructions to be "balanced on the head without any weight on the forearms and fully extended 'up'." Despite adhering scrupulously to the details of the pose and holding it for 45 minutes every morning as instructed, over time she began to feel pain in her face and neck. And the pain got worse.

She reasoned that if she had hurt herself, then her students risked injury as well.

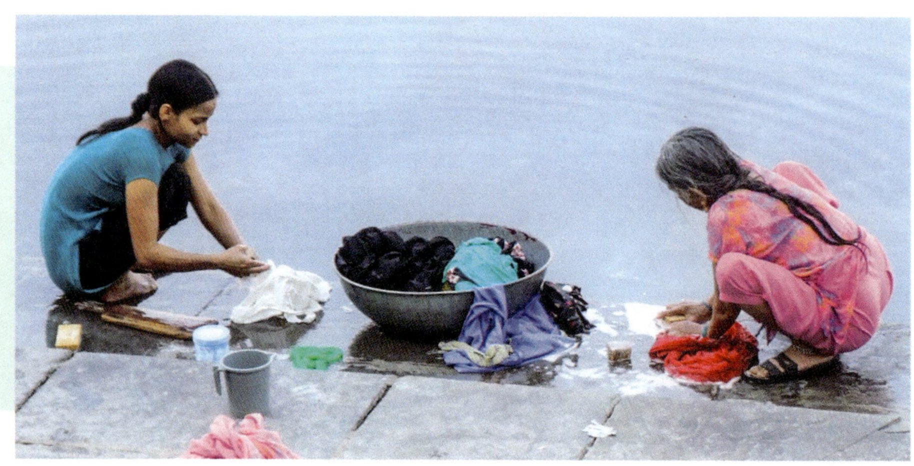

A young woman and her grandmother wash clothes in Bangladesh. Notice the difference in the position of the spine and the opening of the hips. Whose back is more likely to feel tired or strained?

Nöelle hypothesized that standing with weight on her head would take her one step closer to a headstand. If she could find someone who carried the equivalent of their own weight on their head while standing still, they might show her what she was doing wrong in a headstand.

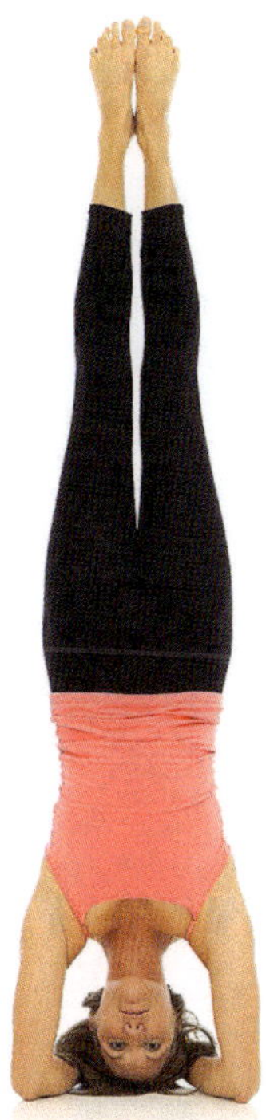

Yoga headstand.

Her research revealed several key findings:

- With rare exception, no one carries as much as their own weight on the head or stays immobile while carrying this weight.
- While carrying, the major joints (shoulders, hips, ankles) are aligned along a vertical axis, which transfers the weight to the heels.
- X-rays of subjects in Burkina Faso and Portugal show the lumbar curvature is always in the same place, right above the sacrum.

These findings became the cornerstone of Nöelle's work.

It turned out that her subjects were aligned in this way whether they carried objects on the head or not. They were naturally upright, moving gracefully and with ease. She noticed a similar posture in much of Setubal's population and called it "Aplomb"—in alignment with gravity as measured by a plumb line. At the Balance Center in the U.S. we call it "Balance."

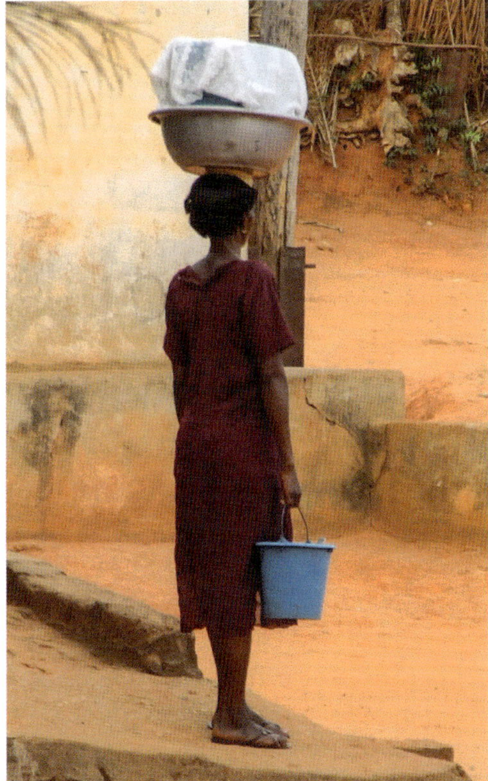

An unhuried woman effortlessly carries a stack of heavy, wet laundry.

Alignment and Gravity

Gravity is the root of lightness; stillness the ruler of movement.

~ Genevieve Brady[7]

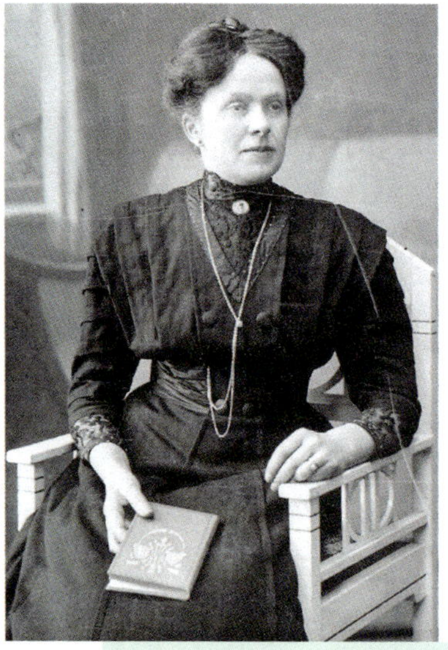
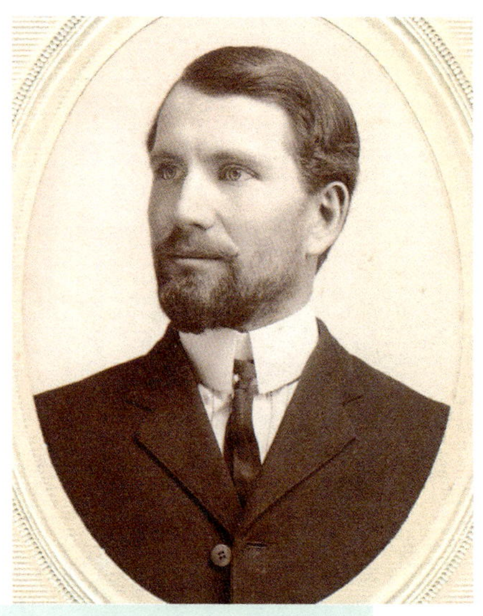

The characteristically erect and sometimes regal look of our ancestors is striking. (Left) The author's grandmother, about 1925. (Right) Unknown man, 1910.

The principles of balanced alignment are apparent to anyone who has ever stacked building blocks or dominoes. Only with precise alignment and exact distribution of weight will the pieces stay in place. The laws of alignment are the laws of gravity; they apply to anything in space, be it a building, boat, or person.

Earth's gravitational pull holds our feet to the ground and attracts our bodies toward the center of the earth in a direction we call vertical. When a wall's verticality is confirmed with a plumb line as true, the wall is perfectly aligned and the building will be solid. When our skeleton is aligned with the universal plumb line, we feel light and stable. Our weight is evenly distributed, and no holding or tensing is required. When this alignment is absent, muscles and joints must compensate. This wastes energy and causes wear and tear on the spine and joints.

Balance refers to the optimal alignment of our bones in space, and an optimal distribution of weight. We all began life in Balance; every healthy child is born in alignment. But industrialization and sedentary lifestyles have altered our habits, undermining the alignment and ease we were born

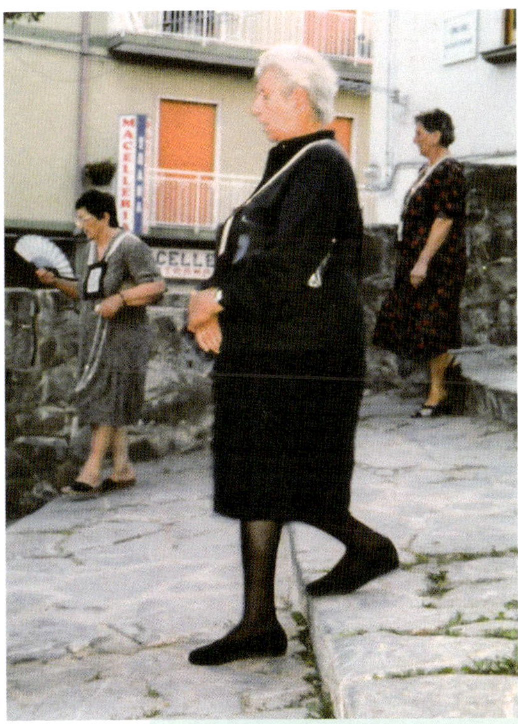

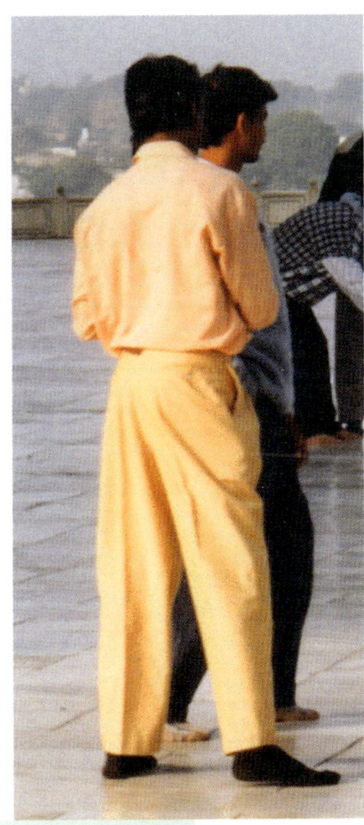

Naturally upright and moving with grace, at any age.

with. And we continue to adapt to the changing demands of today's workplace: less physical activity, more desk work, and more time in our cars, commuting.

Not only did industrialization lead to more sitting, but as people adapted to a changing lifestyle women's fashions became less restricted and formal. In the 1920s it became fashionable to stand with the pelvis pushed forward, which has influenced posture ever since for men and women alike.

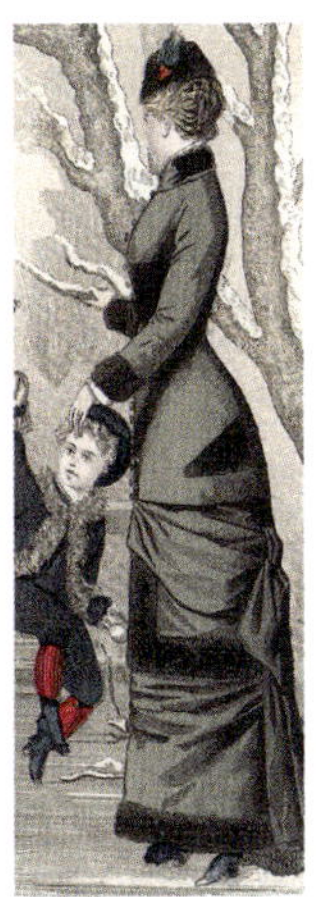

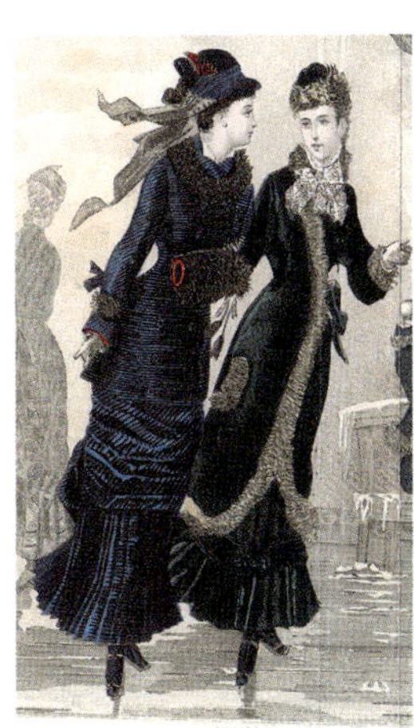

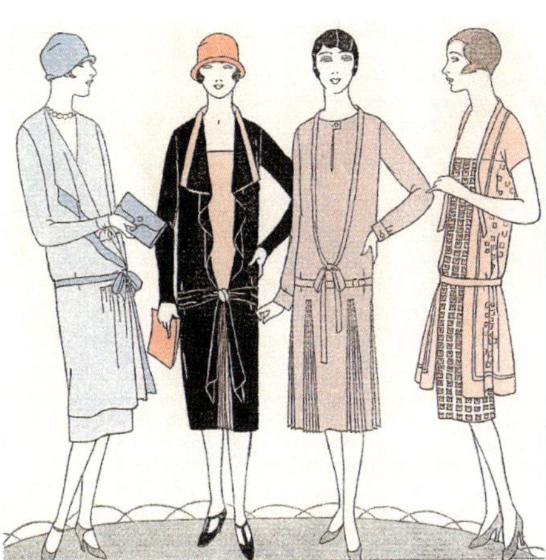

(Left) 1880—Standing upright along a plumb line. (Center) 1880—Maintaining upright alignment while ice skating. (Right) 1924—Disturbing the plumb line by pushing the hips forward.

FASHIONABLE POSTURE

Since they arrived, the 27 South African kids visiting the Traveling School International in Santa Cruz have been getting their ears pierced, bleaching their hair and learning to slouch so that they are now indistinguishable from the locals.

~ "California Dreamin'," *San Jose Mercury News*, March 1996

We now accept discomfort and are hardly aware of it. Women wear high heels regardless of foot pain. Computer screens invite craned necks, and keyboards hurt our wrists. We adapt until we get hurt. Back and neck pain, carpal tunnel syndrome, and hip and knee injuries are epidemic in Western culture.

Depending on how you stand or sit, you are either in a state of struggle or a state of ease, either in conflict with gravity or in harmony with it. When a person is in Balance there is no friction, no resistance to gravity. There is only ease.

The difference is visible in rural India and Africa where people work in the fields, women often with a baby strapped on their back, or walk long distances to carry water. The people are resilient and look graceful. In rural Portugal and France the elderly tend their vegetable gardens straight-backed and with surprising stamina. They are in Balance: solidly placed and stable.

Balance enables people to be comfortable, pain-free, resilient, and graceful at any age. Balance provides a foundation for any activity—sitting, standing, lying down, playing a musical instrument, dancing, gardening, or engaging in sports—whatever you do.

But how can we regain the balance we had as a child? What does it look like? What does it feel like?

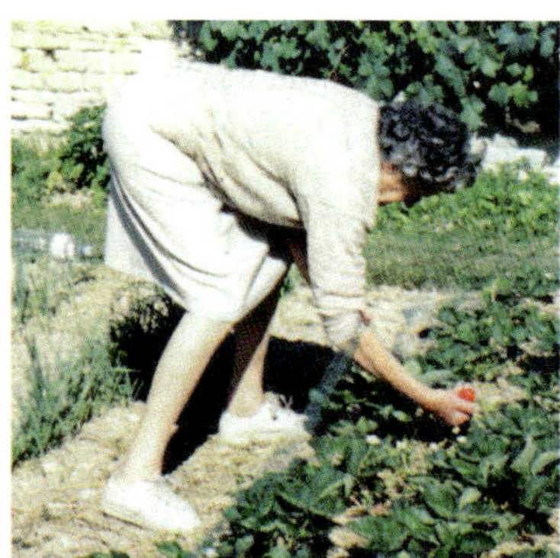

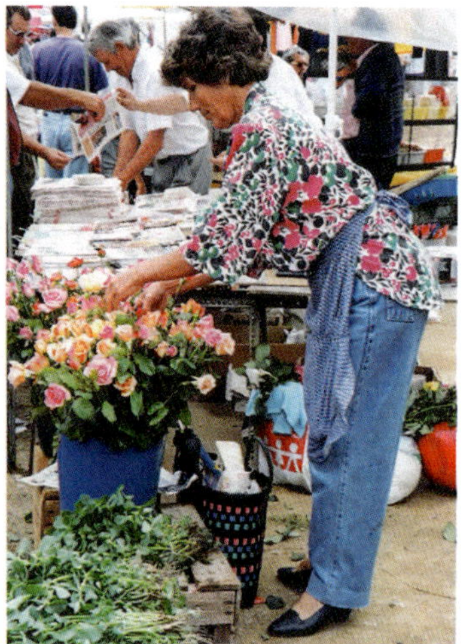

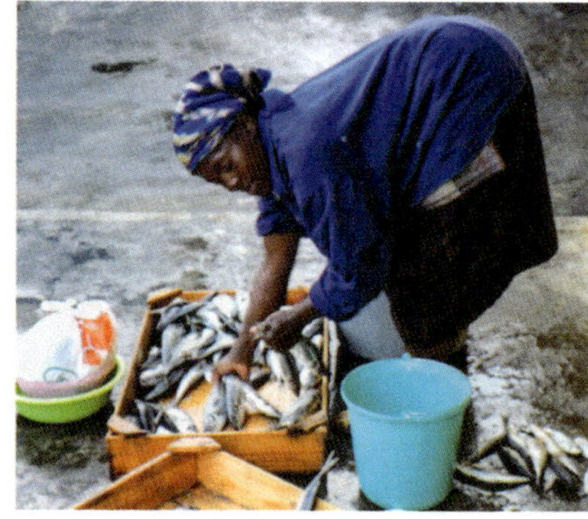

In Balance. A 76-year-old French gardener, a Portuguese flower seller, and a Portuguese fish market vendor.

THE LOOK AND FEEL OF BALANCE

Of the dozens of people who passed only two women walked as they once all did—goddesses is the only word. The rest thumped and clumped and flumped and were clumsy and graceless, just like us. As a girl I used to watch village women walking to the well, one hand held up to steady the cans on their heads, and tried to be like them, but I could not do it.

~ Doris Lessing[8]

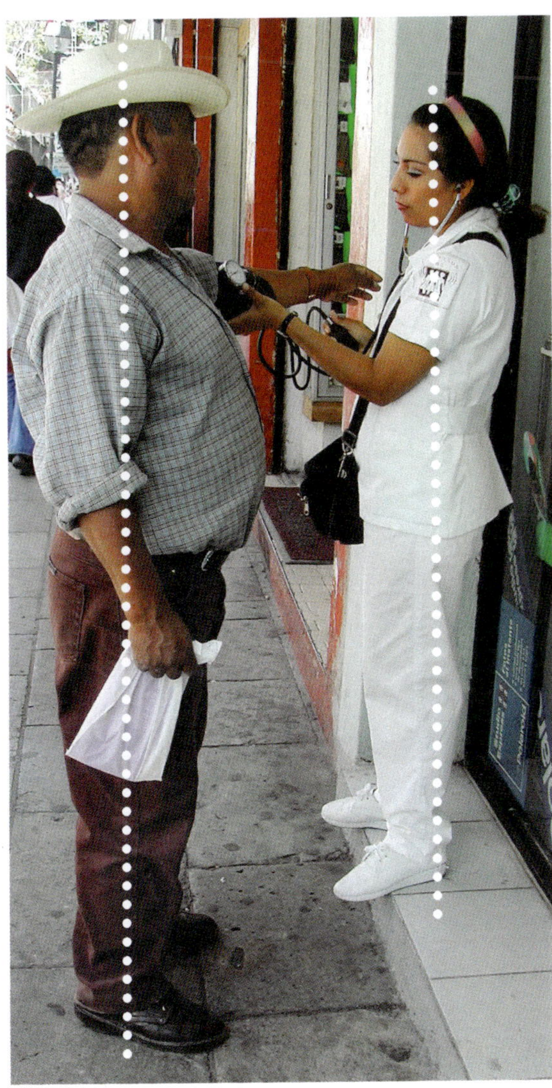

The look of Balance: Upright posture without tension.

Balanced alignment may not be recognizable to you at first. Since most people around us are not in Balance, we must train our eyes by looking at pictures. You will see plenty of images throughout this book of people who are in and out of alignment. You will quickly learn to recognize the difference.

What Does Balance Look Like?

The most obvious characteristic of Balance is an erect posture that looks relaxed. You can see this on the previous page and in the following photos. A person in Balance looks strong and yet at ease.

Being in Balance means that your weight is aligned evenly along a line that extends through your center. We call this line the axis of gravity.

When tension has built up in muscles and joints we no longer follow this line. Patterns of tension and holding fix us in a more or less zigzag pattern. A first step is to relax this tension and *feel* the difference, so that we can move gradually from *holding* ourselves upright to *being* upright.

Who looks more at ease and graceful in the photos on these two pages?

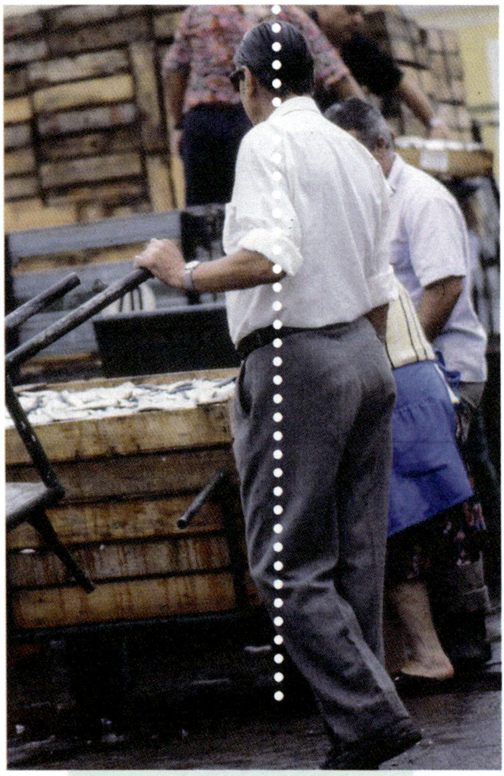

In Balance. Vertical, as measured by a plumb line, without tension.

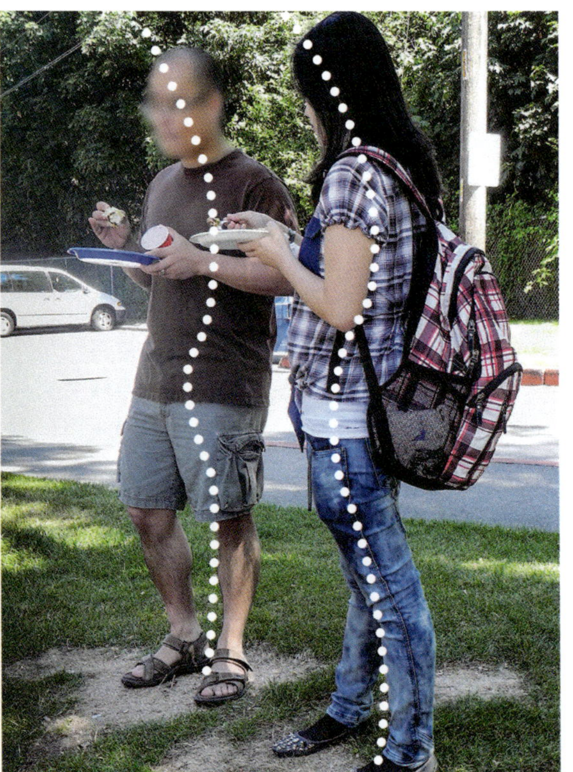

Out of Balance. Zigzag shape with hips forward, knees locked, legs tense.

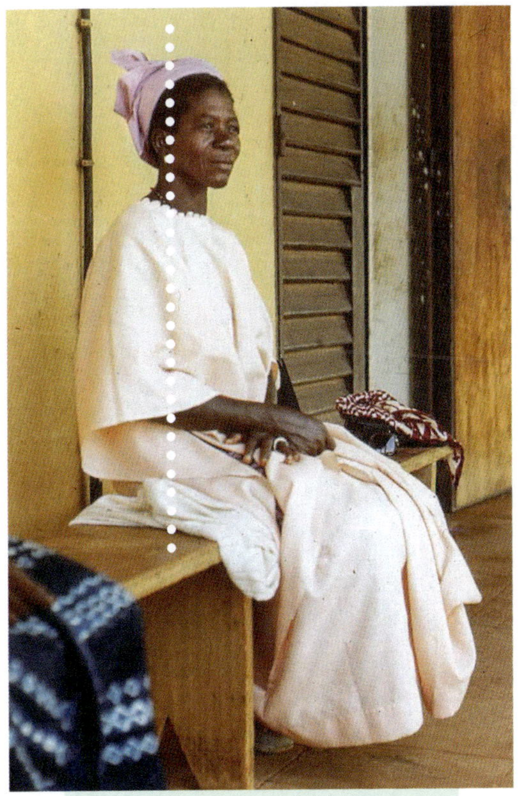

In Balance. Straight spine aligned with head and neck.

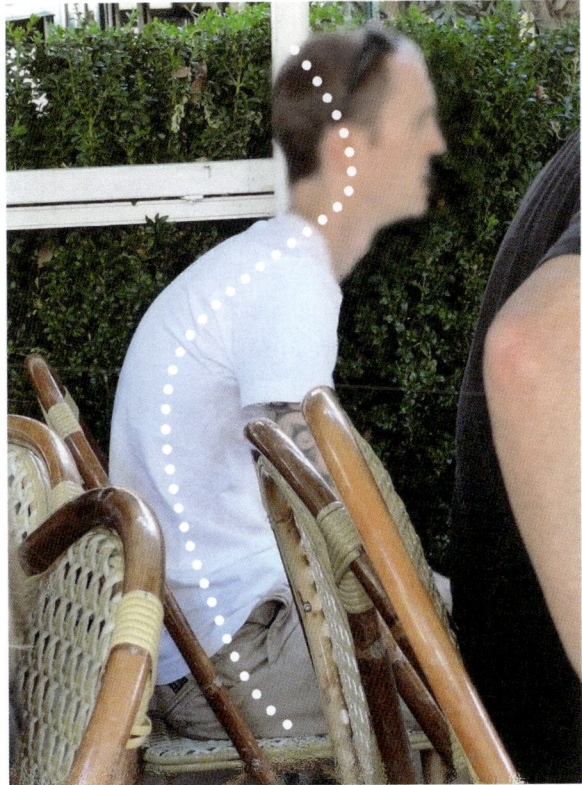

Out of Balance. Rounded spine, arched neck, forward head.

What Does Balance Feel Like?

Nöelle describes living in Balance as "the accurate position of our body in all circumstances of daily life."[9] What is this accurate position?

Suppose that you had to carry a 30-pound basket of laundry on your head. In your current condition your neck would probably collapse immediately. But people who carry weight on their heads for a living—for example, a Portuguese villager who carries laundry every day—counter the weight by lifting up through the whole spine and neck to meet the load.

The direction of up is the axis of gravity, the universal plumb line. People who carry heavy loads on their head every day are obliged to "live on the axis," to follow this line as they lift and lengthen up toward the load. It is the secret of their strength and endurance and it protects them from injury.

You can try this yourself (safely!). Sit on a firm chair, lowering yourself on to the seat as if you were squatting so that your buttocks are well behind you. Put a small weight, such as a book or your keys, on your head. Notice how you have to lift up through your spine and neck to balance the object on your head.

Now take a heavier book and lift the crown of your head to meet the weight as if pushing it away. Begin lifting from your pelvic floor and notice that your whole spine extends. The direction of this lift is your axis. Following this line routinely in all you do is living on the axis.

No stiffening or holding is required; just let your weight settle around the axis. Notice that you cannot do this while holding your belly tense! You must be relaxed first, and then lift. You will feel your belly stretch up along with your spine.

Asking yourself several times during the day, Am I on the axis? will begin to reveal habits of slouching, craning your neck, or lifting your shoulders. It is useful shorthand for teaching yourself to break the habit.

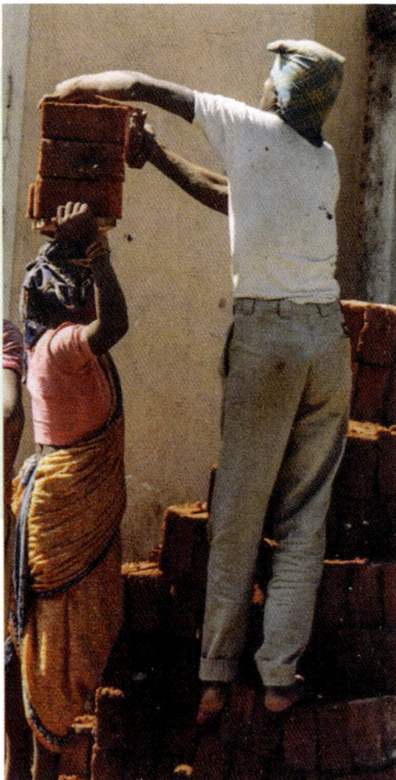

In Balance. Even as she prepares to carry a heavy load of bricks on her head, this woman maintains a vertical alignment and lengthens her spine up toward the bricks. The man lifting the bricks on to her head also maintains this upright alignment.

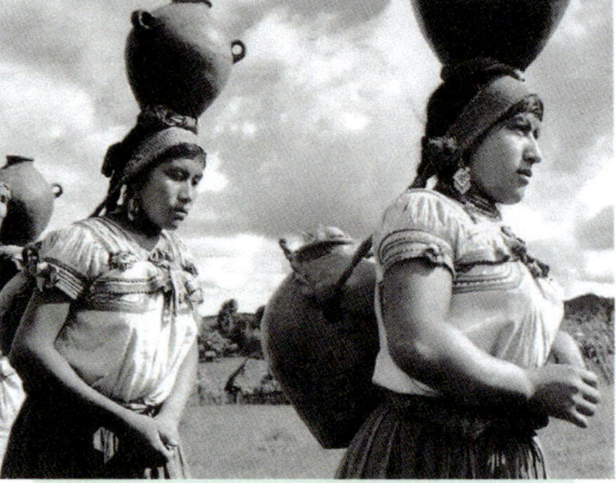

In Balance. These women carry two heavy water jugs at once. One is placed on the crown of the head. The other hangs against the sacrum, held in place with a carrying belt that rests on the front part of the head. The women lengthen up through the spine to meet the weight.

Carrying this much weight without injury is possible only with precise balancing of weight and counterweight—the way it has been done for centuries.

ALIGNING YOUR BONES: FOLLOW THE LINE

Be careful not to carry the shoulders, arms, head and neck in a rigid or stiff posture while walking or exercising.... All the joints should be kept free and limber.

~ Maud Smith Williams[10]

When tension has built up over the years it creates bumps and humps in the spine, tense shoulders, tight muscles, and pain. These tensions shape us into misalignment.

How can you identify where your tension has accumulated?

Face a full-length mirror and draw an imaginary line—the median line or midline—that divides your body down the center. When the two sides are exactly symmetrical, this median line will be aligned with the axis. When they are not, there is work to be done to loosen up tight areas that pull you off center.

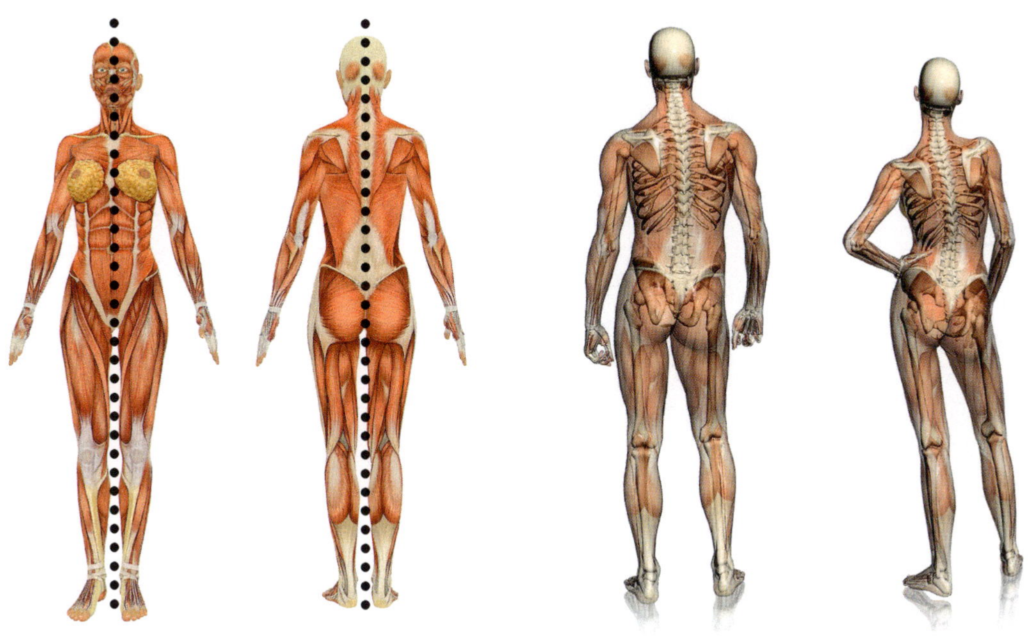

With proper alignment the median line divides the torso into symmetrical halves. When the two sides are no longer symmetrical, the frame is pulled out of alignment.

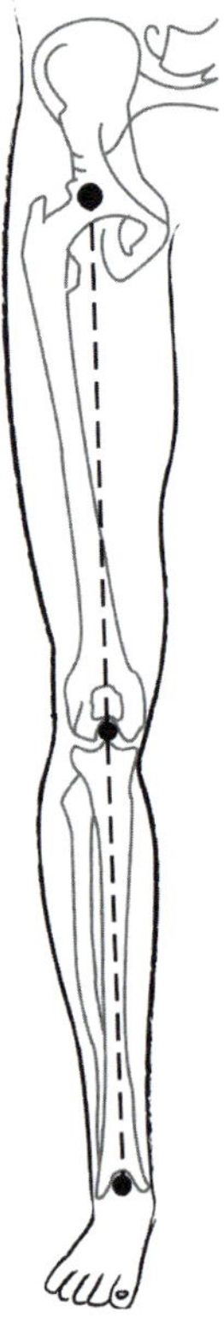

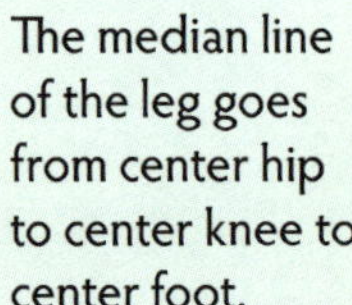

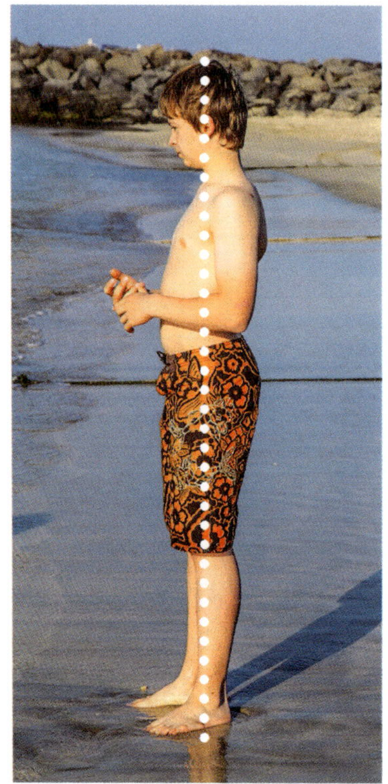

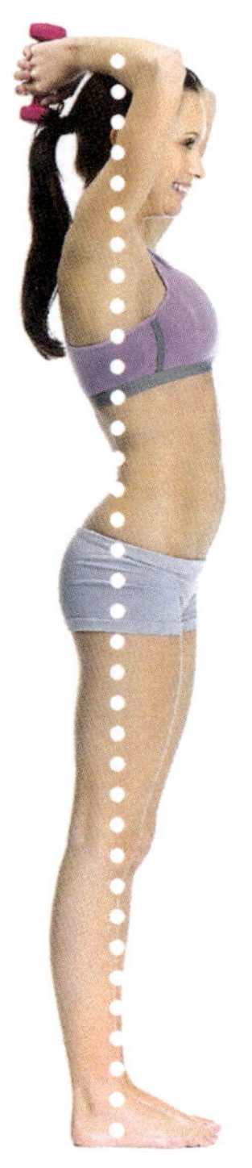

The median line of the leg goes from center hip to center knee to center foot.

In profile you can draw a vertical line from the middle of the head to the heels and that line will pass through the trochanters (at the top of the leg bone where you feel a bony knob, the trochanter bone) and a well-defined natural arch of the spine.

The legs of the boy at left follow this line, but the girl arches her back, stiffens her legs, and locks her knees. He is **in Balance;** she is **out of Balance.**

FOLLOW THE LINE

"Follow the line" is a reminder to keep extending and lengthening the spine in all you do. This is how you learn to live on the axis.

Looking at your alignment in profile, a straight line should pass through your neck, spine, and legs down to your heels. See the contrasting photos on the next page.

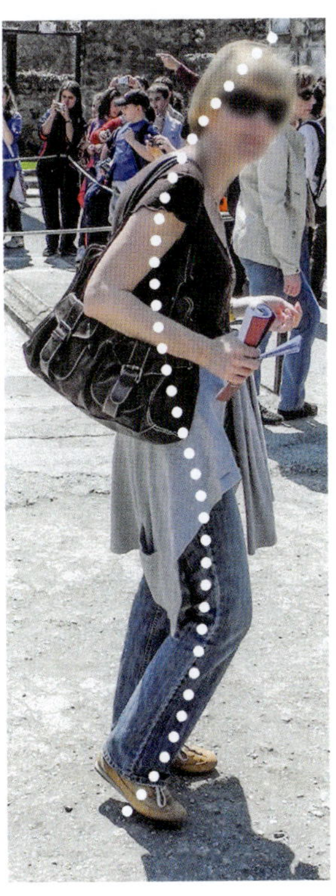

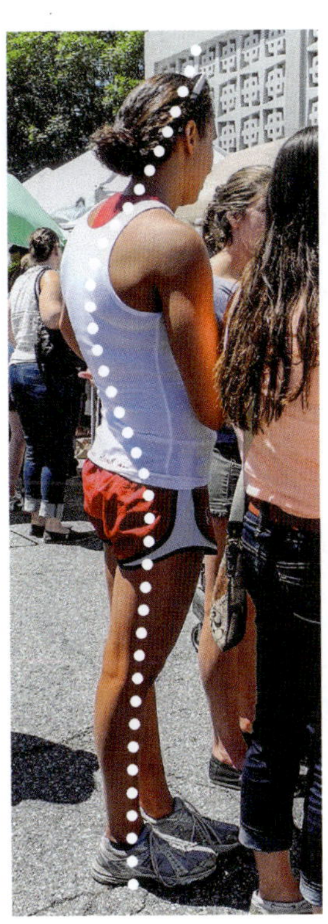

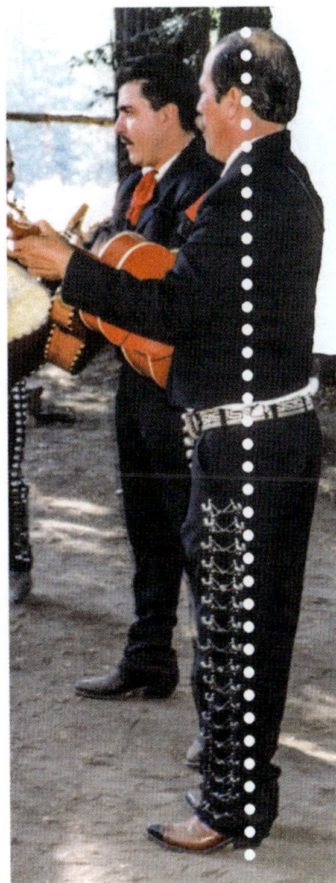

Out of Balance. (Left) Zigzag shape. (Center) Locked knees, pelvis pushed forward, arched midback, and rounded upper back with forward head.

In Balance. (Right) The mariachi player is in perfect alignment. The decoration on the side of his pants is as straight as a plumb line. His back is long and he stands with ease. He lives on the axis.

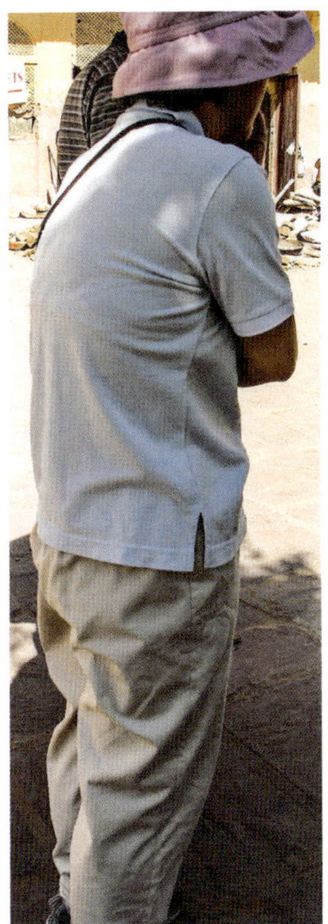

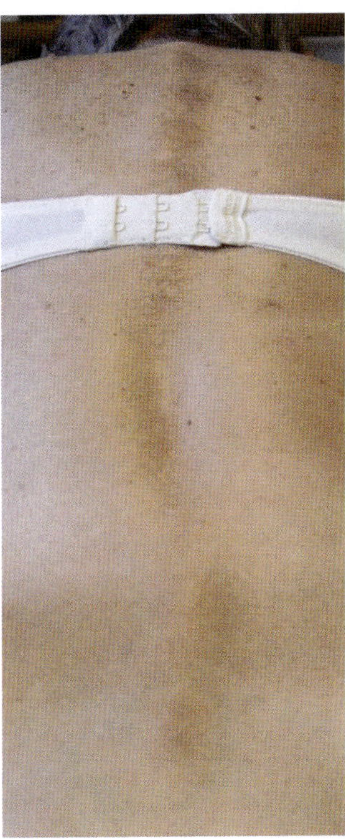

Out of Balance. When the median line is not centered, the vertebrae and joints are vulnerable to mechanical stress due to misalignment of the bones. This leads to osteoarthritis or injury.

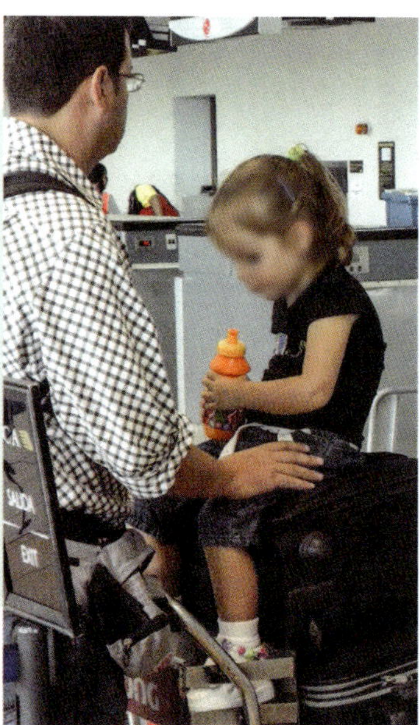

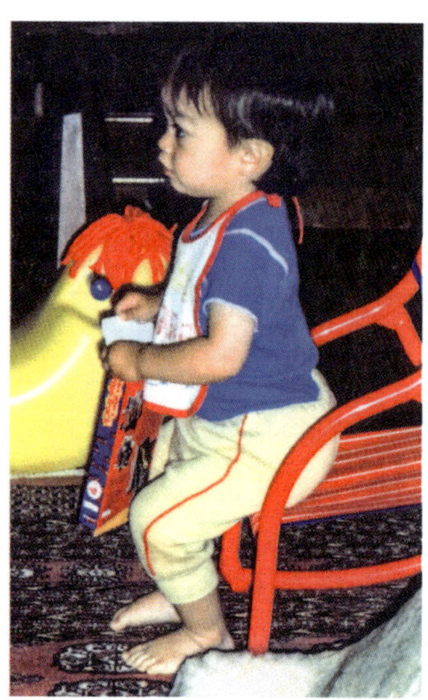

(Left) **Out of Balance.** Habits that create misalignment can start at a very young age. This child has already learned the habit of sitting tail-tucked with a rounded back and compressed organs. She looks old!

(Right) **In Balance.** Notice the difference in the alignment and energy of this child. Until the age of three or four most children are in Balance. After that they begin to change.

CHECK YOUR ALIGNMENT

☑ *Stand facing a full-length mirror. What do you see?*

Are your shoulders or hips uneven, one higher than the other? Do you lean to one side? Do you stand tall, or stooped? Is your head forward? Are your hips pushed forward? Reach around and feel your spine. Are any vertebrae protruding?

☑ *What do you feel?*

Do you feel more weight in one foot than the other? Do you feel tension in your neck, shoulders, or back? Do you feel off-center?

Likewise, evaluate yourself while sitting. Explore, feel, and become aware. Sense how you move and recognize when it is possible to move with ease and when it is not.

When you begin to understand which of your habits interfere with fluid movement and ease, change becomes possible. Examine from the inside out why, where, and how you hold yourself in unnatural or artificial ways. What hurts and when? What tires you?

This awareness will prepare you for the task of aligning your bones. You will also benefit from some understanding of anatomy. The rest of this section explains how the spine, pelvis, and abdominal muscles are critical to balanced alignment.

THE CURVES OF THE SPINE

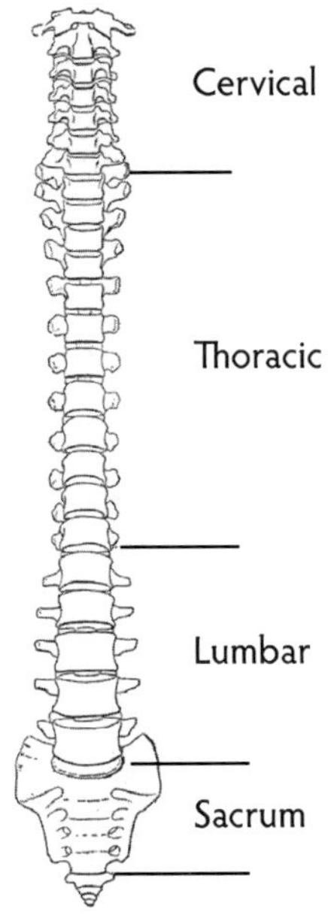

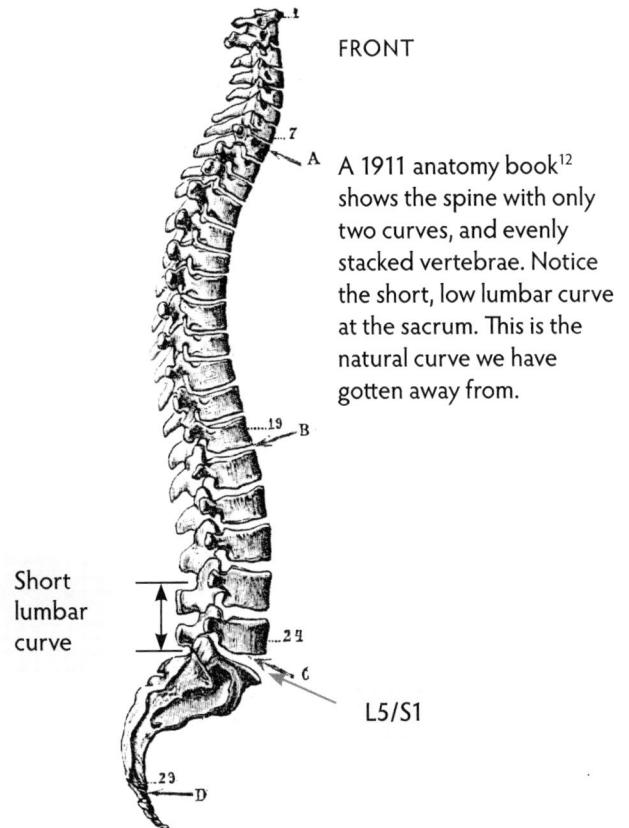

The spine has 24 vertebrae that are grouped top-down as cervical (C1-7), thoracic (T1-12), and lumbar (L1-5), plus 5 fused vertebrae (S1-5) that form the sacrum. Each group forms an opposing curve: the cervical, thoracic, and lumbar curves. The shape of these curves has a direct effect on spine health and general well-being.

Nöelle Perez-Christiaens found that in industrialized countries our spinal curves are deeper and longer today than they were in the past. However, in pre-industrialized countries this is not the case. Close observation and evaluation of X-rays of people who are still in Balance reveal only two curves: a more or less deep lumbar curve and a small thoracic curve. *There is no cervical curve.* The lumbar curvature is deepest where it meets the sacrum, at L5/S1.

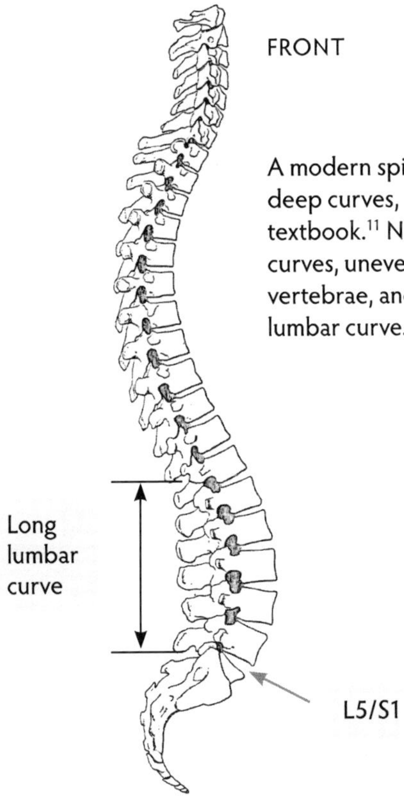

FRONT

A modern spine with long deep curves, from a 1992 textbook.[11] Notice the three curves, unevenly stacked vertebrae, and the long lumbar curve.

Long lumbar curve

L5/S1

FRONT

A 1911 anatomy book[12] shows the spine with only two curves, and evenly stacked vertebrae. Notice the short, low lumbar curve at the sacrum. This is the natural curve we have gotten away from.

Short lumbar curve

L5/S1

The Natural Arch, Where Spine and Sacrum Meet

As evolution transformed the spine from a horizontal to a vertical, upright position, the spine had to bend backward. This was anatomically possible only at the intersection of the spine and sacrum.

Looking at an illustration of the spine, you will notice that the sacrum forms a little shelf, which serves as a plateau for all the vertebrae stacked above it. The angle of the sacrum plus the shape of the first two vertebrae above it gave the spine its ability to curve from horizontal to upright.

Only here, at L4 and L5, are the lumbar vertebrae shaped to bend the spine. The natural lumbar curvature that begins at this spot is what Balance teachers call the natural arch. It encompasses vertebrae S1, L5, and L4.

The natural arch is the only place where the spine is designed to bend backward safely. Overriding this anatomical design and routinely bending back at the waist instead of at the natural arch is a cause of considerable pain and injury, especially in yoga and exercise, where back-bending postures are common.

The natural arch at L5/S1 is the hinge that allows the spine to bend backward safely. This baby's spine begins to rise from that point.

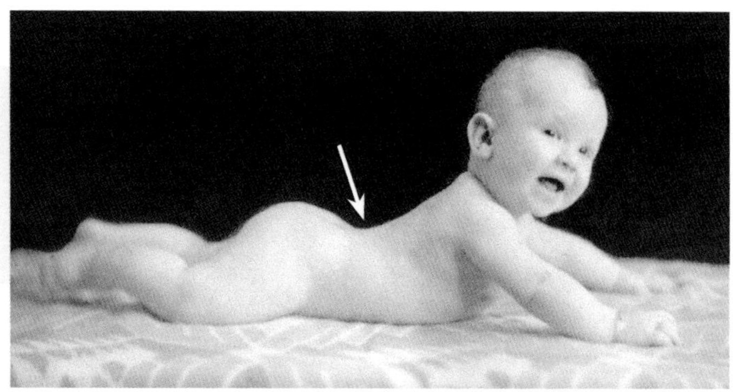

This is a crucial point and the core of Nöelle Perez-Christiaens' research. As she discovered, our spines today tend to have a long "false" lumbar curve—a hollow, tense back. This is due to our habit of lifting the chest to straighten up, which arches the back and squeezes the lumbar disks.

The low lumbar spine is the most frequently injured part of the back and is exactly where the shape of the spine differs most between people who are in and out of Balance. The deeper and longer the lumbar curve, the more unevenly the vertebrae above it are stacked, thus squeezing the disks. One secret to preventing pain is to avoid arching the back. Always bend back at the natural arch, never at the waist.

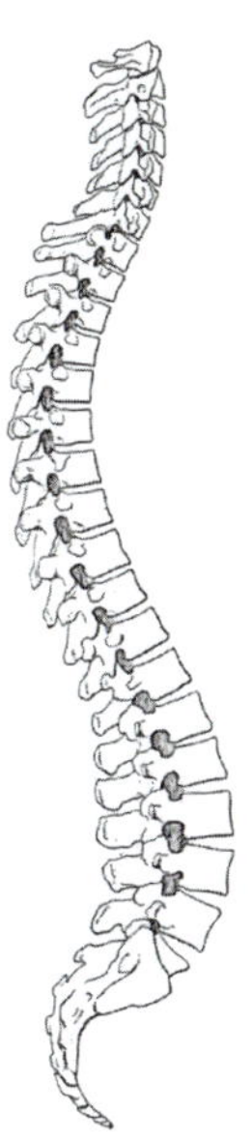

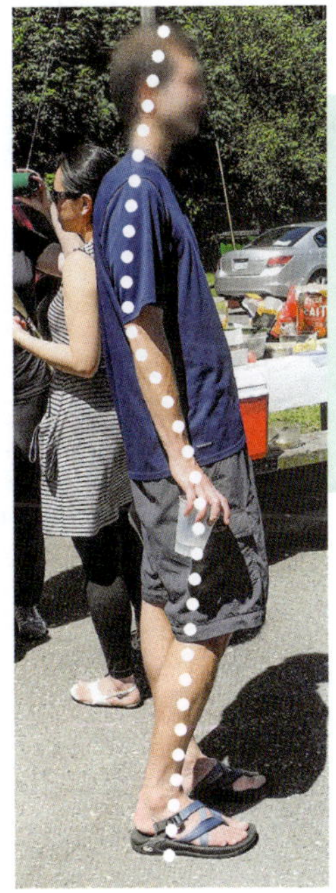

Out of Balance. This man is not vertically aligned because his pelvis is thrust forward as he stands. To compensate and to remain stable, he has to lean backward. The result is an overly curved spine, very common in Western cultures. Notice the drop of the buttocks.

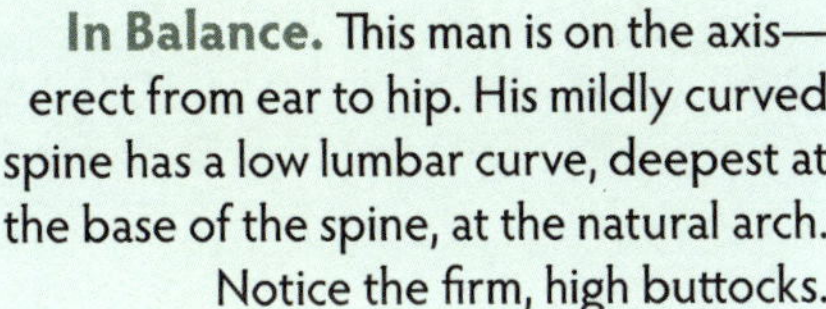

In Balance. This man is on the axis—erect from ear to hip. His mildly curved spine has a low lumbar curve, deepest at the base of the spine, at the natural arch. Notice the firm, high buttocks.

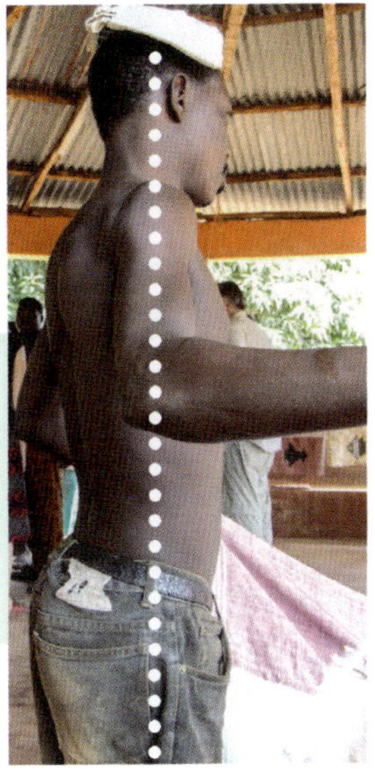

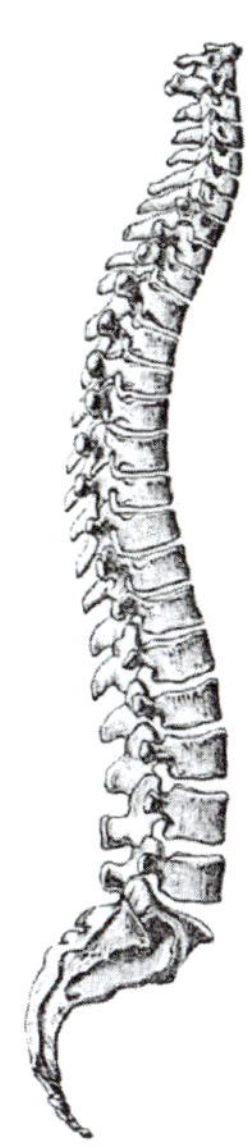

Out of Balance. Straightening up by lifting the ribs and creating a hollow back is dangerous and can cause injury. The lift should begin at the natural arch.

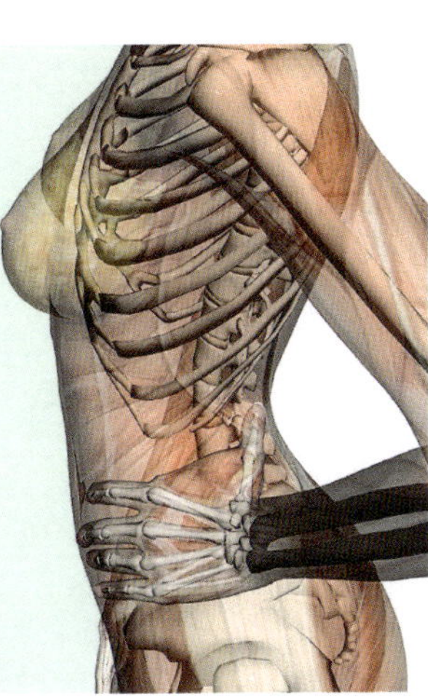

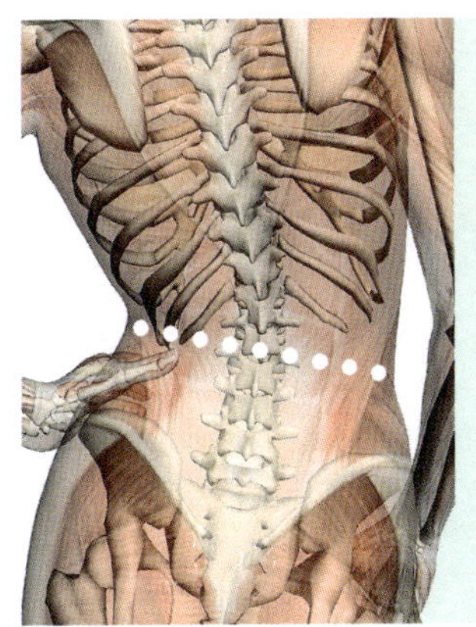

Out of Balance. It is important to lengthen from evenly placed (horizontal) hips to stack the vertebrae and prevent friction in the spine.

In a healthy back, an even groove begins at the sacrum—at the natural arch. There are no bumps or hollows, no vertebrae that poke out or go deeply in. The muscles along the spine (the erector spinae) look and feel relaxed.

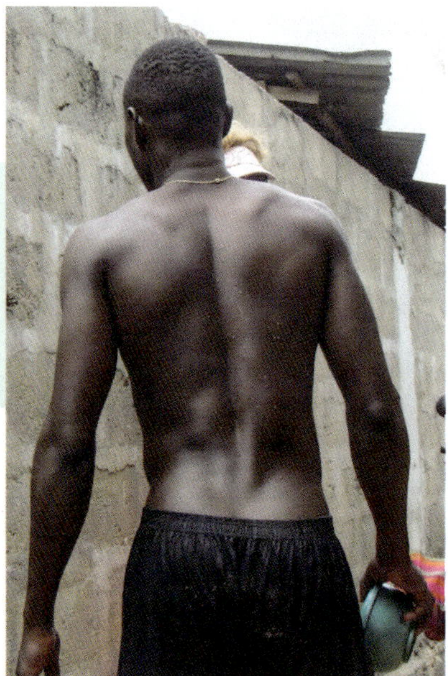

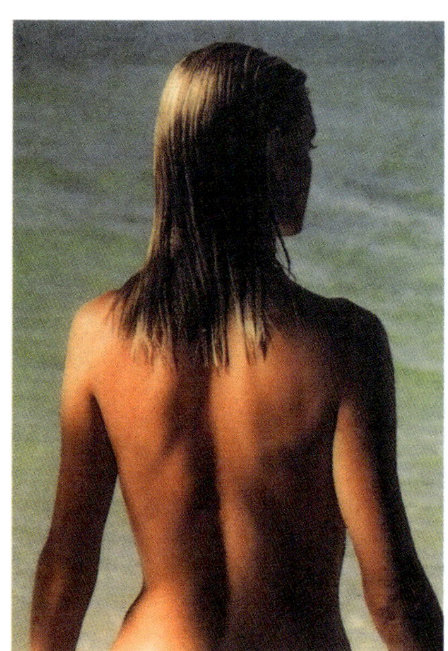

In Balance. Examples of a healthy spine with an even groove that begins exactly at the sacrum, at the natural arch.

Locating Your Natural Arch

To find the natural arch on yourself, circle your hands around your hip bones so that the thumbs meet in back. Then slide your thumbs down one to two inches. That is the approximate location of your natural arch, where the lumbar spine meets the sacrum.

The key to Balance is to *straighten up and lengthen from this point*—never by lifting the chest! Only then do the front and back of your trunk work in tandem. Only then will your vertebrae be stacked evenly so that your spine can lengthen. Straightening up by lifting the chest, as many of us were taught, is a common cause of injury.

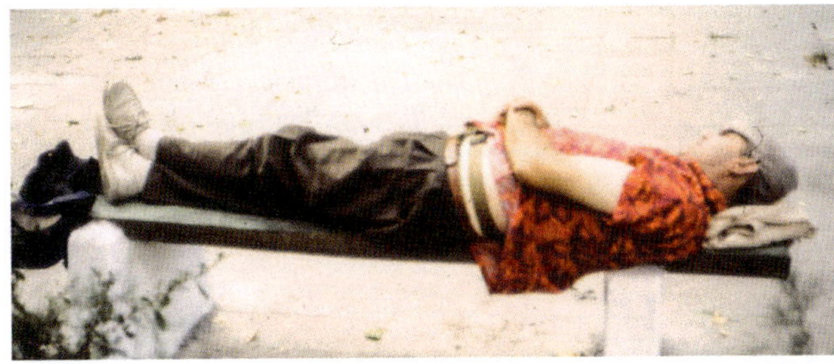

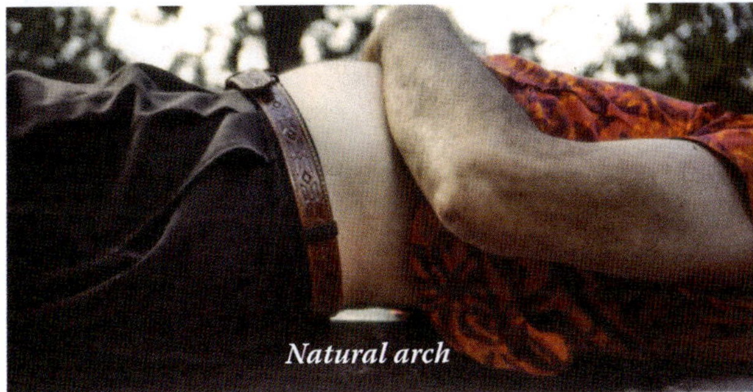

In Balance. Here Miguel is asleep on a bench. His back is flat on the bench except for a small rise where light comes through the space that is created. This is the natural arch, right above the sacrum.

The more we recover our true lumbar curve, the less our upper back will round and the more our neck will also straighten. This is a chain reaction that begins at the natural arch, where spine and sacrum meet. Extension of the spine starts there.

This brings us to the pelvis and its role in spine health.

THE PELVIS

The position of the pelvis is the most important and also the most subtle and difficult part of reestablishing alignment and Balance. You will need hands-on instruction from a qualified teacher to fully understand and benefit from these principles.

The pelvis resembles a bowl formed by the pubic bone in front, the hip bones at the sides, and the sacrum in the back. The sacrum is the tail end of the spine.

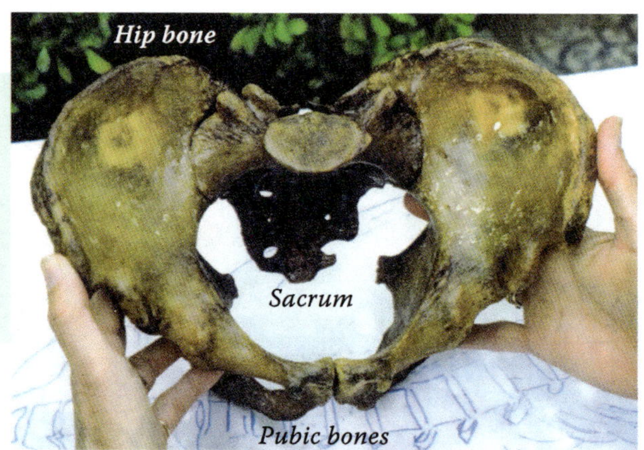

The ability to straighten up from the natural arch is determined by the position of the pelvis:

- Out of Balance: When the front of the pelvis is lifted up, it flattens the natural arch. You are forced to lean back and lift the chest, creating a hollow back (a false natural arch). From there it is impossible to extend the spine in a straight line.
- In Balance: When the front of the pelvis rotates downward, the natural arch keeps its shape and enables the spine to lengthen in a straight line from that point.

See the photos on the next page.

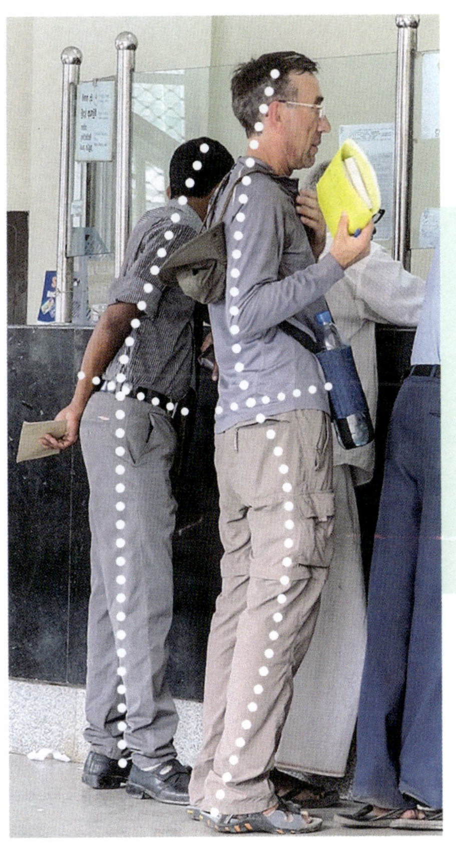

The pelvis determines the shape of your spine. The man at left is **in Balance.** His downward-sloping belt indicates his pelvis is rotated forward and down.

The man holding the yellow folder is **out of Balance.** His pelvis is lifted in front and hangs down in back in a tail-tucked position. He must lean back to stay upright, which makes it impossible for him to have a straight spine. Notice the zigzag shape from heels to knees to hips and up his spine. Notice also the difference in the shape of both men's buttocks.

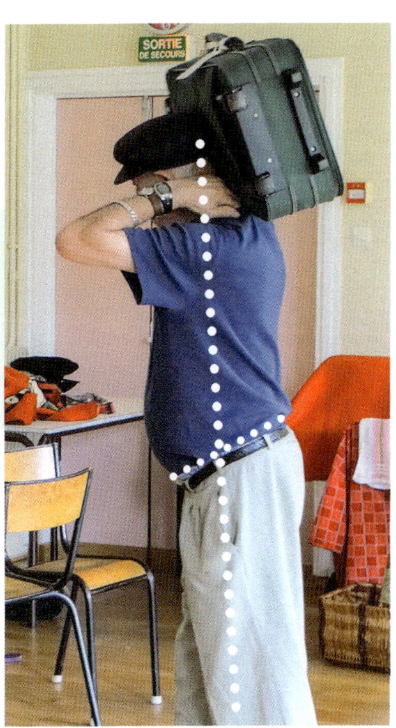

In Balance. This photo of Miguel illustrates the pronounced downward slope of his pelvis, following the belt line. His spine adheres to an invisible plumb line.

It is important to understand that rotating the pelvis down in front requires mobility in the low back (at L5/S1), in the hip joints, and in the sacroiliac joints. *Rotation should never be forced.*

To feel the downward rotation, gently let weight settle in the front of the pelvis. You are likely to notice tension in the groin near your hip joints, and in your low back. With time and practice you will learn to increase mobility in these areas and allow the pelvis to find its true position (rotated down).

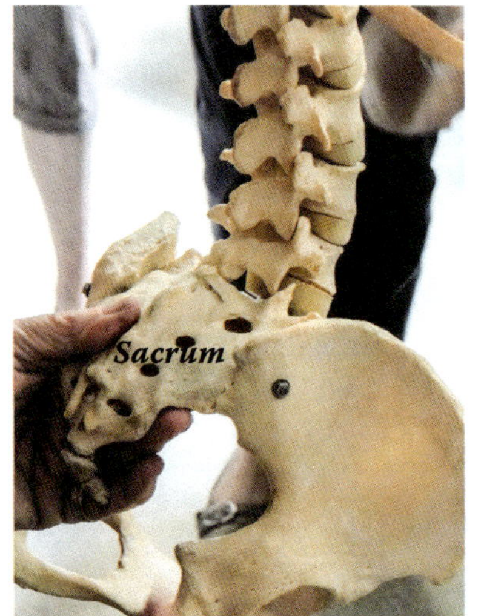

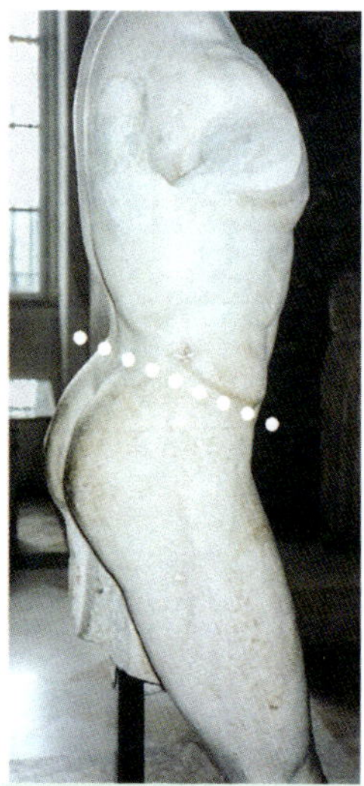

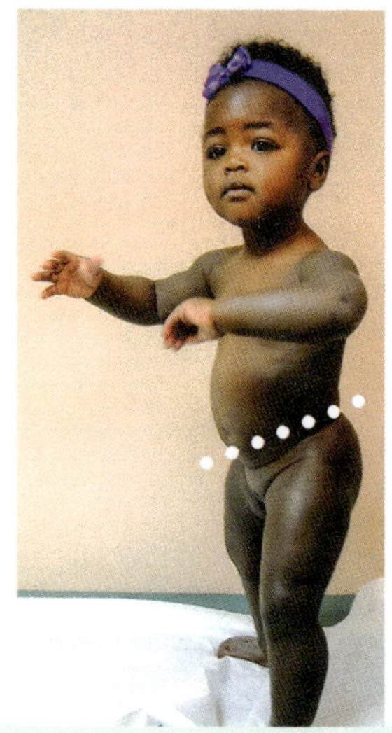

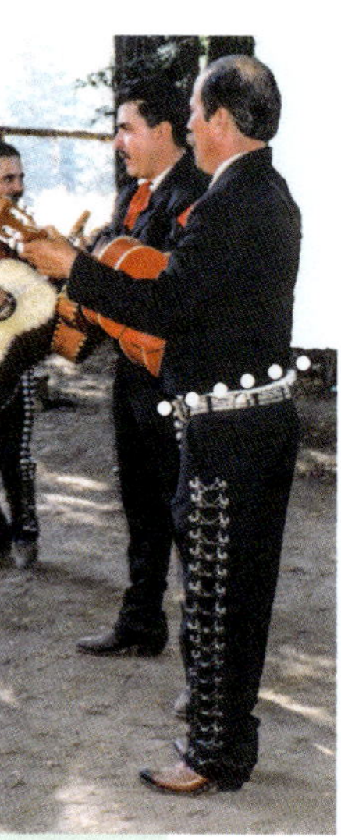

In Balance. The triangular sacrum bone at the base of the spine angles back when the pelvis is rotated down (lowered) in front. Compare the statue and the toddler with the mariachi player: A belt placed on either one, following the edge of the hipline (the pelvis), would slope down in front like the mariachi's belt.

Feeling the Pelvis

The following steps will help you become acquainted with the position of the pelvis and where to place the weight.

First, you need to locate your sitting bones:

- Sit on a firm surface (a wooden or folding chair or bench), lowering yourself onto the seat as if you were squatting. This places your buttocks well behind you. The seat should be high enough to let your thighs slope down slightly from your hip joints, and low enough so your feet are flat on the floor. (If you have long legs, bend your knees and slide your feet underneath you or elevate the seat with a firm blanket or pillow.)
- Lean forward, then slide your fingers under your buttocks and sit on them. You will feel knob-like bones pressing on your hands. These are your sitting bones (ischial tuberosities), two curved bones that extend from the base of the pelvis. These are at the back of the pelvis and very close to the tailbone (*coccyx*), which is at the end of your spine. To feel them more distinctly, rock side to side or back to front.

Next, feel the mobility of your pelvis:

- Put your hands on your hips and gently drop the front of your pelvis (your pubic bone) down toward the seat until you feel weight there. Your pelvis is now rotated forward. Return to your beginning position. Do this a few times and feel the mobility of your pelvis in the up-and-down movement of the hip bones under your hands.

Finally, feel the current position of your pelvis:

- **If you feel your buttocks under you but no bone,** your front pelvis (pubic bone) is lifted and your back pelvis (sacrum) collapses under you. Your weight is behind your sitting bones. Your natural arch is dangerously compressed. Your back rounds significantly.
- **If you feel the sitting bones as knobs under you,** your front pelvis (pubic bone) is somewhat lifted and your back pelvis (sacrum) is compressed. Your weight is on your sitting bones. Your lower back arches at your waist if you try to sit straight.
- **If you feel pressure on your pubic bone,** your front pelvis is lowered and rotated forward and your back pelvis (sacrum) is weight-free. Your weight is on your pubic bone. You are sitting comfortably erect, upright from your natural arch.

This illustration from the Smithsonian archives shows a back view of the spine with minimal curvature and a clearly defined natural arch at the base, between the sacrum and spine. Notice the pubic bone; this is where your weight should rest.

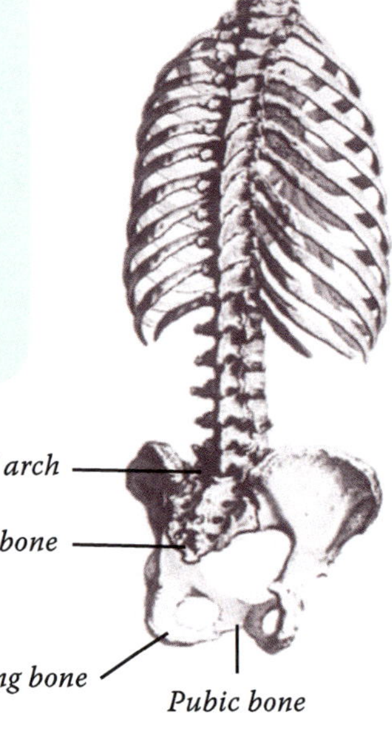

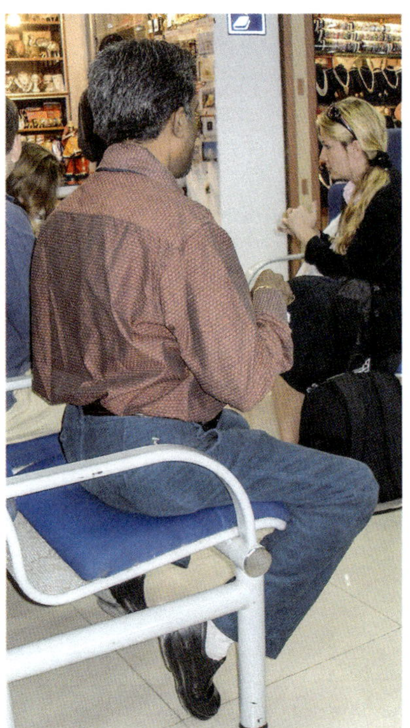

In Balance. This man sits on his pubic bone, at ease and with a straight spine. The front of the pelvis is rotated downward on the chair seat. His spine matches the one at left.

Sitting comfortably erect starts with the position of the pelvis. Gradually you will learn to shift your weight from the sitting bones farther to the front of your pelvis. This takes practice. A teacher can be helpful.

With this new pelvic position you will probably feel tightness in your low back. To relieve it you need to learn to use your abdominal muscles properly. The next section explains how.

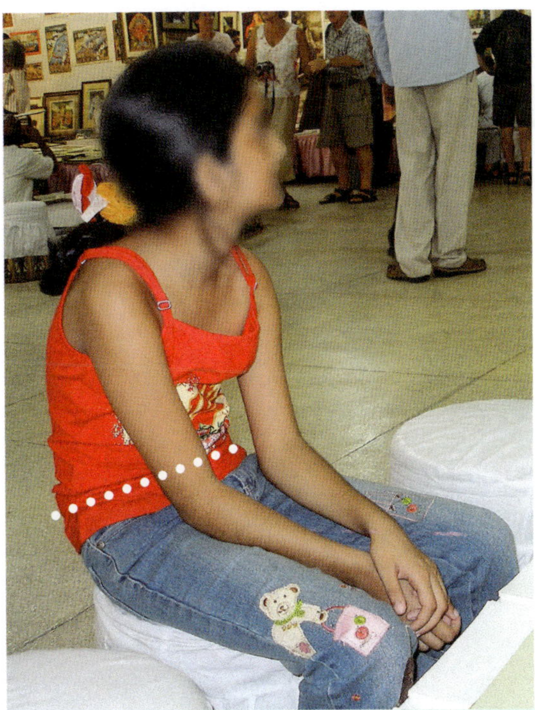

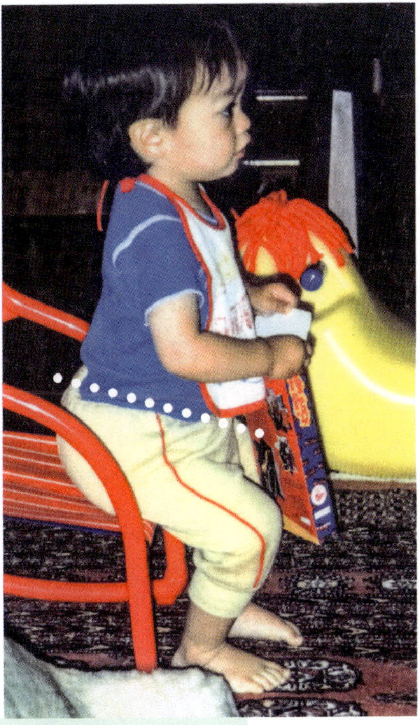

Where is the weight? (Left) **Out of Balance.** The pubic bone is lifted, compressing the back of the pelvis and rounding the back. The girl's weight is well behind the sitting bones, on the tailbone. To sit up "straight" with her pelvis in this position, she has to lift her chest and arch her back.

(Right) **In Balance.** The pelvis is rotated down and forward between the legs, and the weight is on the pubic bone. The spine is erect all the way up from the natural arch. Habits are formed early in life!

FEELING THE SENSATION OF WEIGHT

Alignment and distribution of weight are the cornerstones of Balance. The sensation of weight is unfamiliar to most of us as we start on the road to Balance. We know the word but not the experience of feeling weight. Feeling your weight is a checkpoint that you can use again and again to discover alignment.

THE CORSELET

To properly support the pelvis position just described, you will need to use the muscles of your "inner corset," or what Aplomb and Balance teachers refer to as the *corselet* (pronounced kor-se-LAY).

A well-aligned spine is an extended spine supported in front by the abdominal muscles between the rib cage and pelvis, and in back by the muscles of the spine.

These muscles are fundamental in keeping us aligned and upright. They protect the spine by keeping it extended just enough to prevent undue pressure on any one disk. When the abdominal muscles are weak, the back muscles dominate and pull the spine out of alignment.

The abdominals cannot work properly when you are slumped, slouched, or curved in the wrong places.

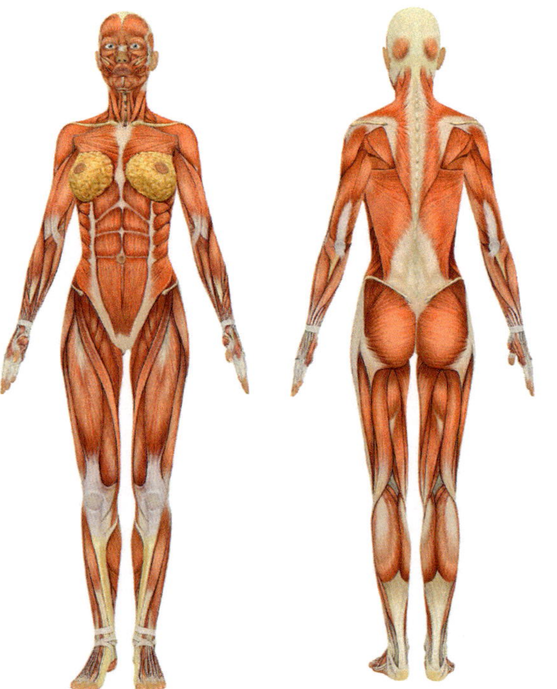

◀ Anatomy of our built-in corset: The abdominal muscles fill the area between rib cage and pelvis, front, sides, and back. The muscle fibers run in lateral, horizontal, and diagonal directions. The muscles are paired, left and right, and must work in symmetry.

▶ This profile view shows the shape of our inner corset, from the pubic bone to the breast bone and wrapping around the sides. When we slouch, bend from the waist, or arch the back, these muscles cannot support an upright trunk, and they weaken from disuse.

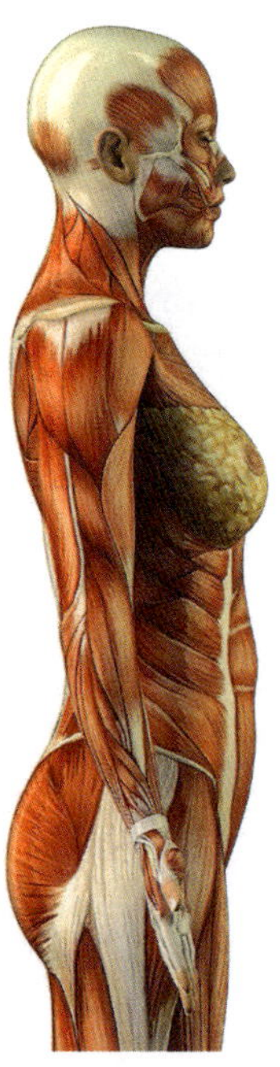

To maintain the habit of a long spine, European women used to wear a stiff bodice, sometimes with whalebone stays, as inner or outer wear. This fabric garment wrapped around the rib cage, harness-like, and closed in front below the breasts. Commonly called a corselet (French for small corset), its purpose was to keep the spine straight.

The corselet was not a corset worn to constrict the waistline for the sake of fashion. When it was in use (until the early 1900s), people were still naturally upright and the corselet was tailored to their shape; it felt snug and comfortable. Women today would not be able to fit into this type of garment without great effort and discomfort because their posture is so misaligned.

To regain an upright bearing without resorting to a structured garment, we need to rediscover our abdominals, the built-in corselet that is tailored to our shape.

THE CORSELET AS GARMENT

The corselet is not to be confused with the constraining, harmful corsets of Victorian times. A corselet is a snug bodice, often with stays, laced in front but not so tight that it interferes with breathing or circulation. To cover the same area, men often wore a similar garment in the shape of a wide, fabric belt wrapped around in several layers to stay warm or for support during physically demanding tasks. This garment is still worn today by bullfighters, for example, as part of their traditional costume.

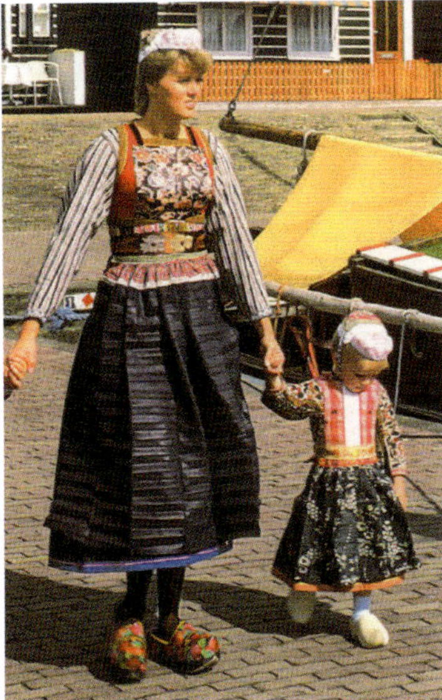

This traditional Dutch costume is still worn today for special occasions. A harness-like corselet wraps around the rib cage, shoulders, and back. Children wear a similar garment.

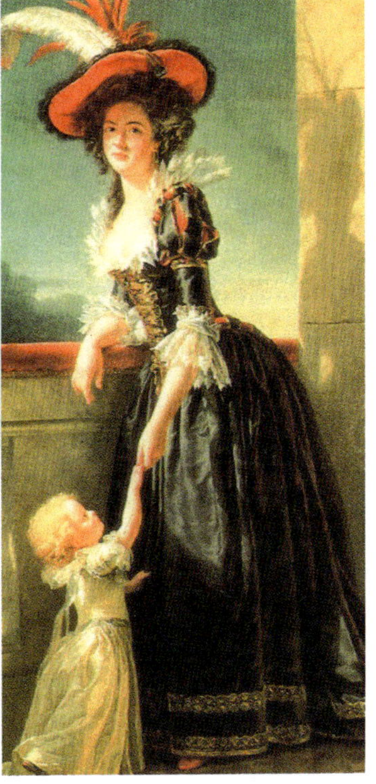

This restrictive corset was worn to change a woman's shape to conform to fashion.

Notice how the corselet on this French statue is laced in front, wrapping below the breasts, and covers most of the back. The fit is snug and was designed to be comfortable.

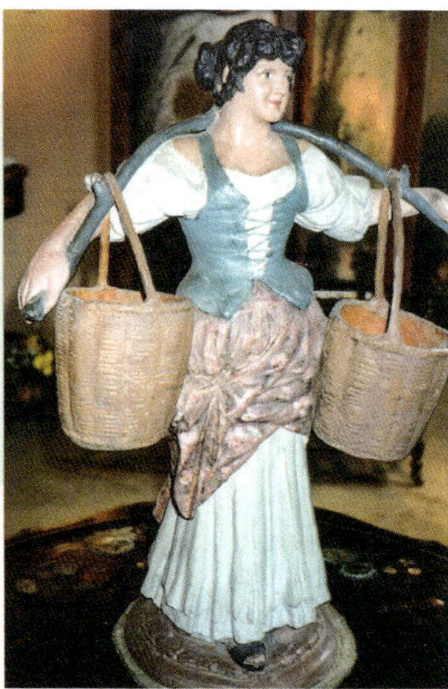

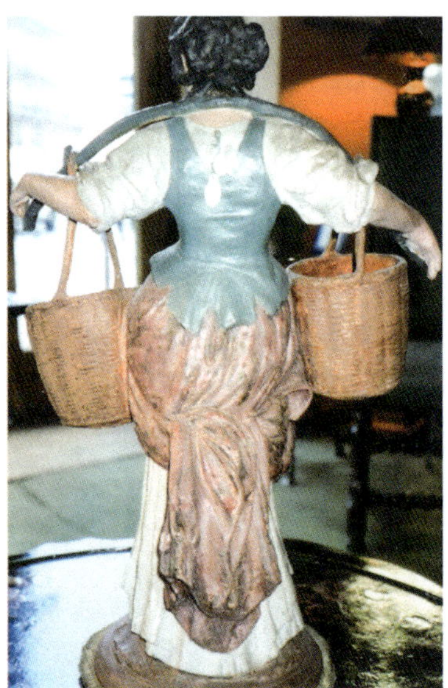

Engaging Your Corselet

To become aligned with gravity we use the concept of the corselet as a reminder to engage the abdominals to lift and straighten the spine.

Become familiar with how this feels:

- Observe how you normally sit upright. You probably lift your rib cage in front to look straight. If so, your back is tense and arched.
- Now imagine lacing a corselet in front: Pull the two sides together with your hands, pressing down on your ribs. You may feel your back soften, and the tension release.
- Now, to straighten up, do not lift the ribs and arch your back. Instead, lift from your low belly and follow the spine up all the way through your neck in a straight line. Can you feel how you begin to stack your vertebrae without lifting your ribs?

Engaging your corselet in this way engages your abdominals to lift and straighten your spine. This extension gives you a feeling of solidity, just as a corselet would.

Before you practice this, it is important to relax. Most of us have learned to sit up straight by lifting the chest and arching the back. If in addition you tighten your stomach to have a flat abdomen, then there is plenty of tension to release before you do anything else. Only a relaxed stomach can stretch upward. Only a released spine can extend. Undoing of muscle tension is essential.

In short, to engage the corselet, lift front and back simultaneously, from your pubic bone in front and your natural arch in back, up the spine. If your back follows this line, you will feel a lengthening all the way up to your head.

If you were carrying something on your head, you would have to do this lifting action continuously to keep the spine aligned and protect it from compression. With balanced alignment your spine supports this action very well, as the stacked disks cushion the vertebrae.

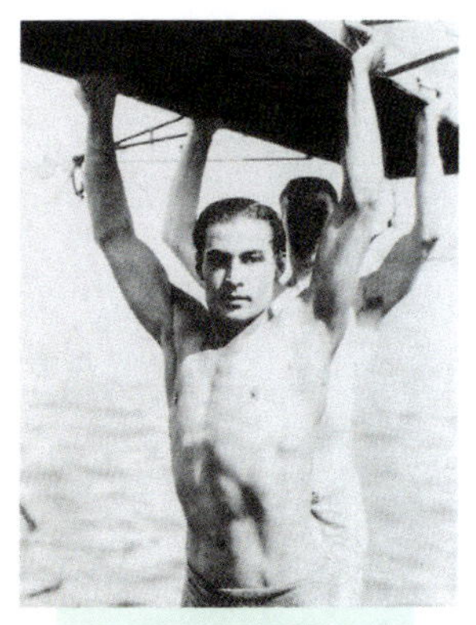

In Balance. Only a relaxed stomach can stretch upward.

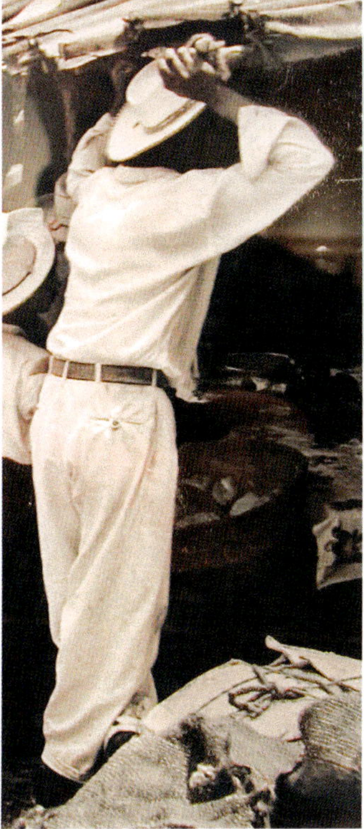

In Balance. Try to lengthen your spine in the same position as this Mexican man does, with your buttocks behind you and without arching your back. Then relax as he does.

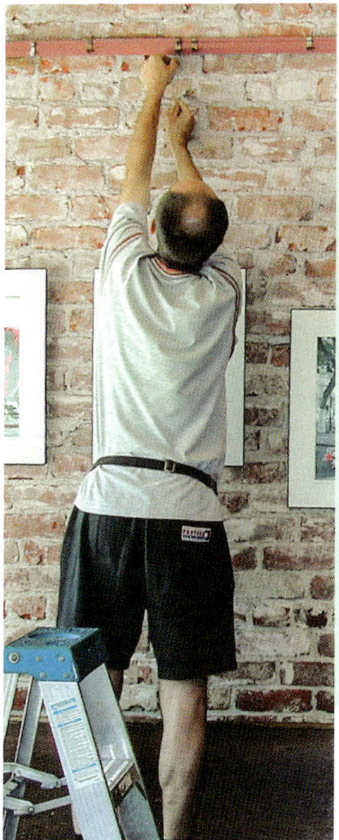

In Balance. In daily life there are many opportunities to practice engaging the corselet. This man is a beautiful example of lengthening from the natural arch. Notice how his hips stay stable (his belt is horizontal) and his legs are solidly planted. He reaches up by lengthening evenly on both sides of the spine (notice the folds of his shirt). His shoulders stay down.

EXTENSION: THE SECRET OF A STRAIGHT SPINE

Extend **1.** *To open or straighten (something) out; unbend.* **2.** *To stretch or spread (something) out to greater or fullest length.*

A secret to relaxing your back is to extend and straighten your spine to its fullest length, so that the disks are not compressed and can cushion the vertebrae as intended.

It is important to experience extension as an opening, a lengthening, or a stretching that creates space in the joints and the spine. At first, when you tell yourself to extend, you will respond instinctively by using the muscles that are easiest to manipulate, while tensing others that you have habitually underused.

Over time and with practice you will learn to stretch both the front and back of your torso evenly. This will feel different from what you are accustomed to. Only when the major bones and joints are in alignment does it become possible to extend and feel length and lightness. It is the quality of your stretch that will lead to the feeling of lightness. There can be no lightness without extension.

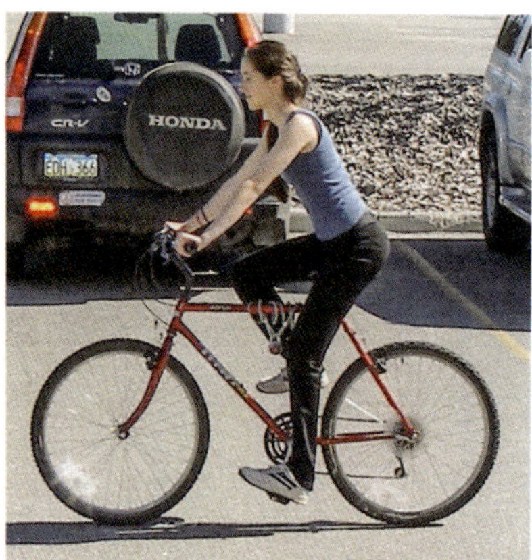

In Balance. The pelvis is rotated down between the legs, which allows extension from the natural arch up through the neck.

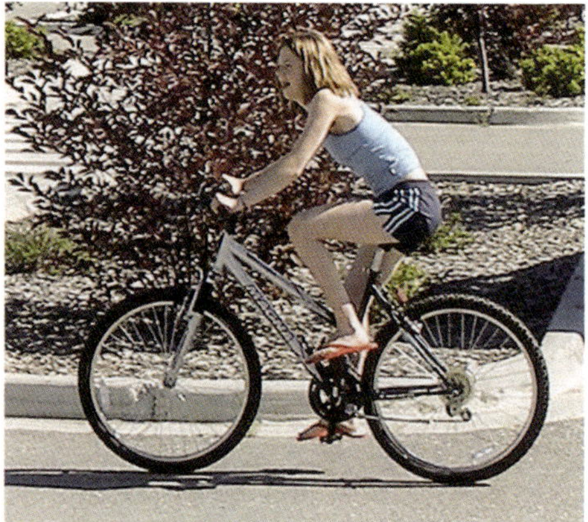

Out of Balance. The pelvis is lifted in front, which rounds the natural arch and low lumbar spine, making extension impossible. Notice the arched neck as a consequence of the forward slope of the upper back and shoulders.

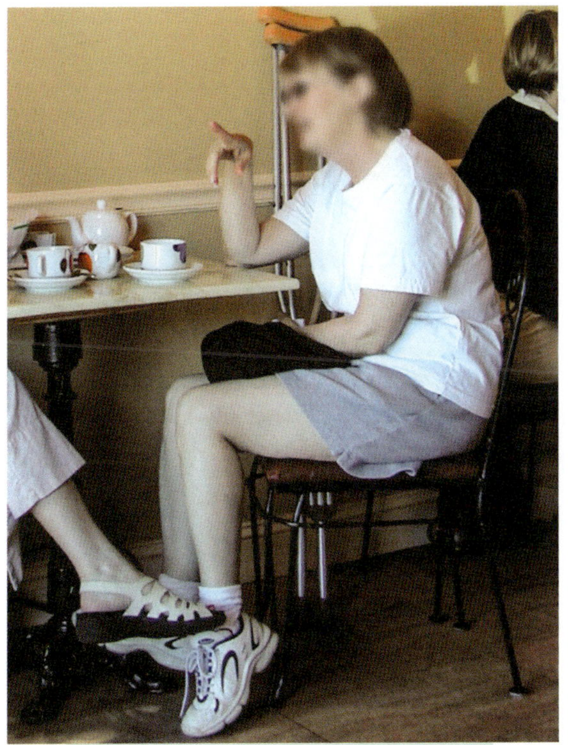

Out of Balance. A shortened spine: The chest is collapsed, the ribs are pressing down on the organs, and the back is rounded. This is the opposite of length and extension.

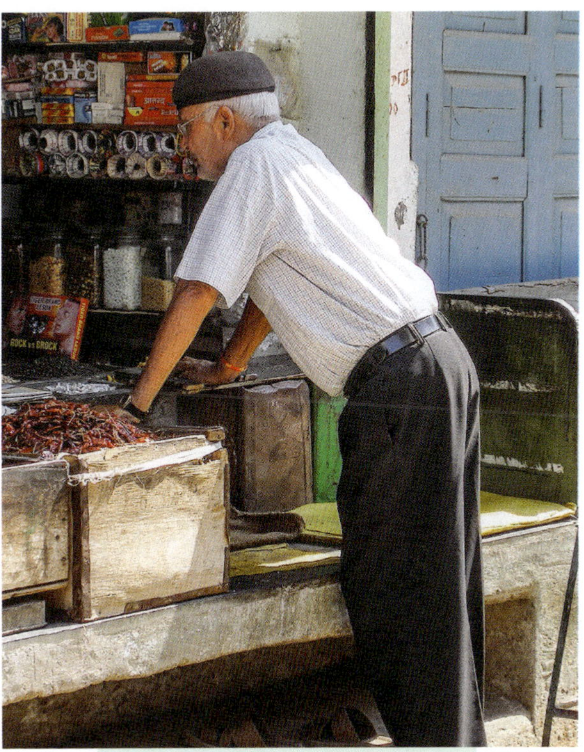

In Balance. Compare this man's back with the bicyclist on the facing page to see the similarity in position of the pelvis and spine.

Extension is elongation. It is the opposite of collapsing on yourself (letting your chest drop and your back round), which squeezes the abdominal organs, affects breathing, and stresses the spine.

An extended spine is a habit, not something to do when you happen to think of it. In the beginning you must practice all day long. This is an excellent form of exercise.

Part 2

PRACTICING BALANCE IN EVERYDAY LIFE

Yoga aims for complete awareness in everything you do.

~ B. K. S. Iyengar[13]

Bending from the hips with a flat back is the best thing you can do to maintain a healthy spine.

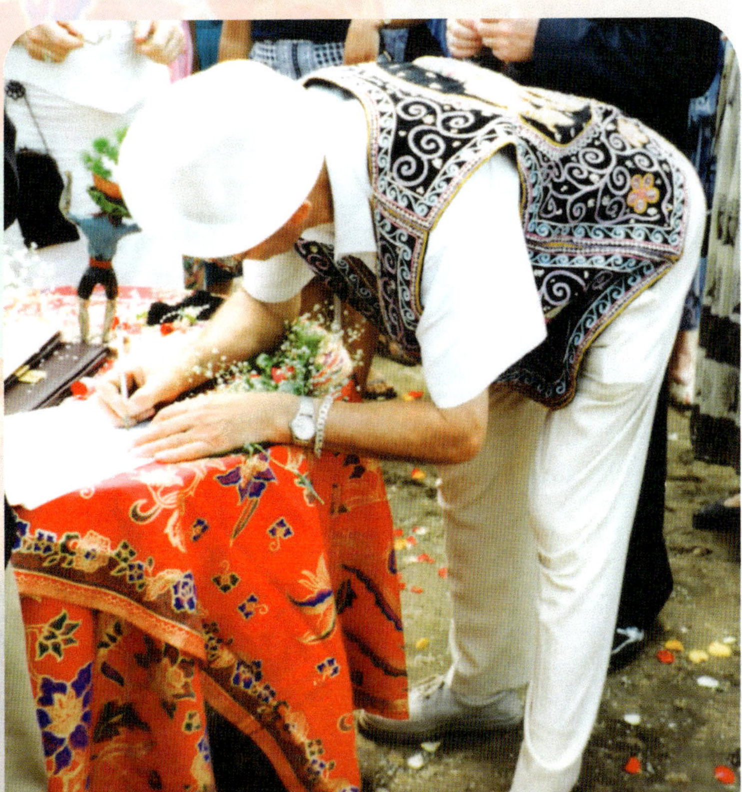

TRANSFORMING DAILY ACTIVITIES INTO YOGA

Nöelle Perez-Christiaens says that Iyengar's description of yoga as "complete awareness" motivated her to leave her yoga studio and transform into yoga "everything I had to do in a more than overloaded life."[14]

As you begin to move with greater awareness, you will discover there are similarities between elementary yoga poses and your daily activities. Standing, bending, walking, lying down, and lifting all make the same demands on you that a yoga pose would. The common element is alignment of the pelvis and the spine.

With attention you will become aware of how pain-inducing habits can be changed and thus relieve your pain. The rewards for your efforts go beyond pain relief, and include youthful poise, vibrant energy, and graceful aging. You begin to feel in charge of your own health.

Every person's body is different, imprinted with the habits and injuries of a lifetime. As you begin exploring Balance, you will benefit greatly from working with an instructor. This person's eyes and hands can skillfully guide you, especially in the beginning, on the path to ease and comfort.

In Part 2 you will learn how to:

- Sit comfortably on a chair with and without back support
- Align your shoulders, head, and neck to prevent strain
- Get up from and recline on a chair
- Sit in your car to drive
- Stand in Balance
- Bend, lift, and carry safely and without strain
- Walk in Balance
- Lie down so you can rest and sleep comfortably

SITTING IN BALANCE

Sitting is about relaxing (passive) instead of arching (active). Your task is to eliminate any surplus activity and to do only what is needed. The unnatural/excessive arch in your back disappears as soon as you relax and your pelvis finds its natural place. You feel weight settle at the pubic bone.

~ Nöelle Perez-Christiaens[15]

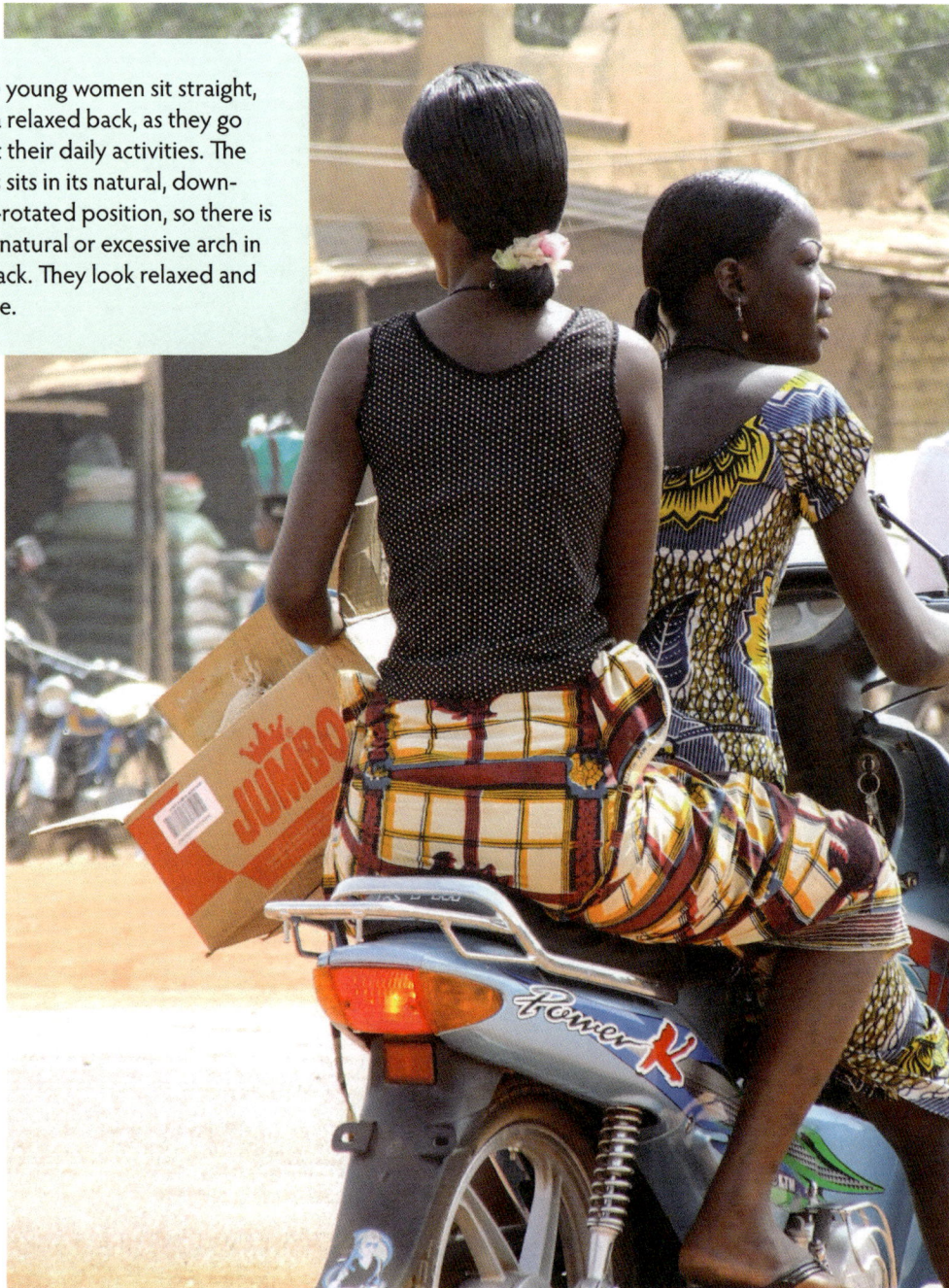

These young women sit straight, with a relaxed back, as they go about their daily activities. The pelvis sits in its natural, downward-rotated position, so there is no unnatural or excessive arch in the back. They look relaxed and at ease.

Positioning Your Pelvis

Most of us spend many hours a day sitting: to eat, nap, relax, watch TV, and even to participate in sports such as kayaking or horseback riding.

Sitting can be perfectly comfortable, safe, and pain-free. It is *how* you sit that makes the difference. The secret is in the position of your pelvis.

As you learned in Part 1, when you sit with your pelvis angled up in front (the pubic bone lifted), your weight rests on your tailbone—on the back of the pelvis—and your spine rounds at your natural arch. This creates tension and compression in the vertebrae. When your pelvis rotates down in front, the weight of your trunk is on your pubic bone—the front of the pelvis. This allows your spine to lengthen. The position of your pelvis determines the shape of your spine. To protect the natural arch, the position of the pelvis is critical.

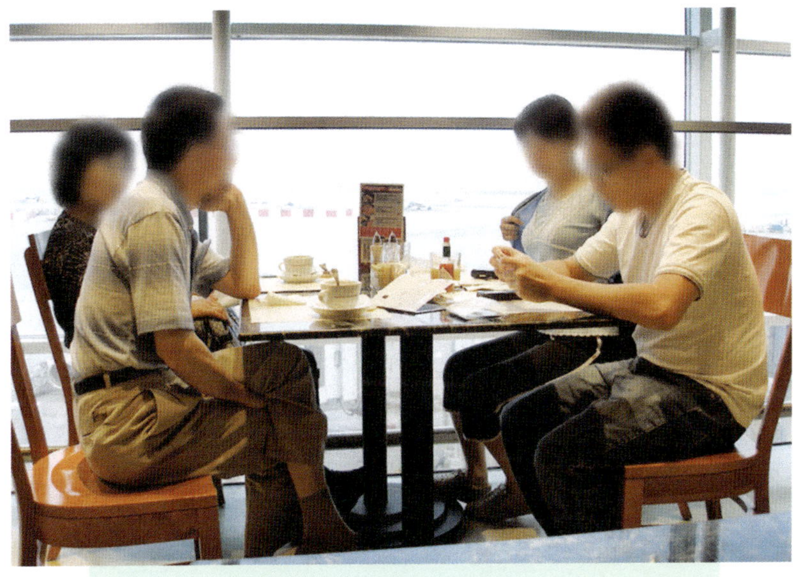

Out of Balance. The rounded shape we all know so well—tucking the pelvis and sitting on the tailbone.

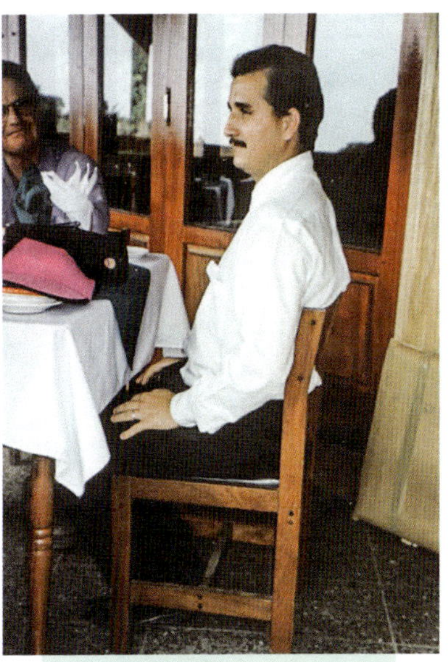

In Balance. Comfortably upright, weight resting on the pubic bone—the front of the pelvis.

Most people sit as shown in the left photo above—on the back of their sitting bones. Simply rotating the pelvis so that the weight rests on the front, on the pubic bone, makes all the difference in the world. Once you learn to sit this way, without strain, you will find that you can sit comfortably on any flat surface.

Sit in a straight-backed chair that is deep enough to accommodate most of the length of your thighs. The height of the seat is optimal when your feet can rest flat on the floor so that your knees are not higher than your hip sockets, and your thighs slope down a little. Tall people may need to fold their legs underneath or alongside the chair to achieve this slope.

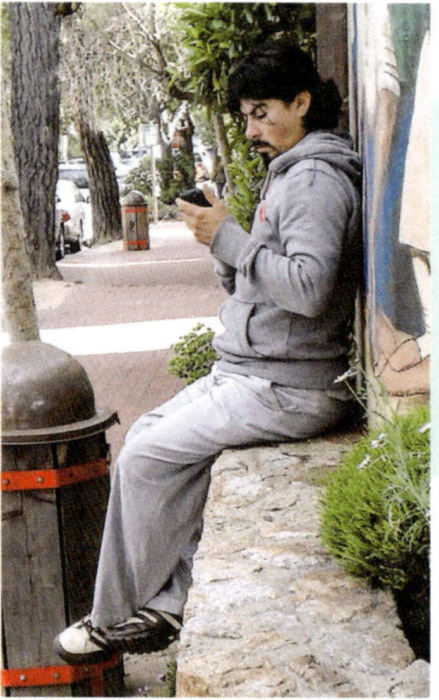

In Balance. This young man has found comfort even on a stone ledge. He slid to the back of the available space so his pelvis is placed well under him. His thighs slope down, which makes pelvic rotation easier, but they are not fully supported. He compensates by resting his feet lightly against the wall.

Sitting with Back Support

HOW TO PRACTICE

FIG

Imagine a fig leaf covering the pubic area of a Greek statue. Use this concept as a reminder to position your pelvis.

"Fig" is a verb. To fig means to lower your pubic bone down and back between your legs, so the weight is on the front of your pelvis.

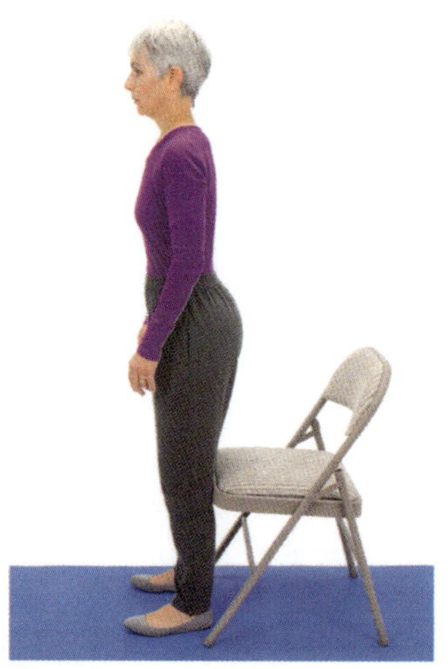

Figure 1

- Stand close to the seat of a chair.

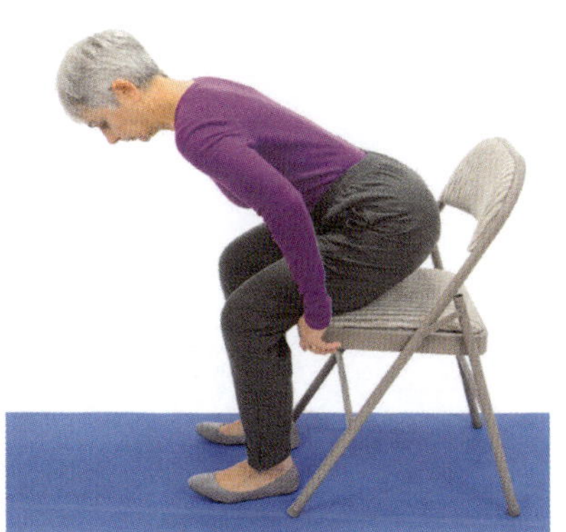

Figure 2

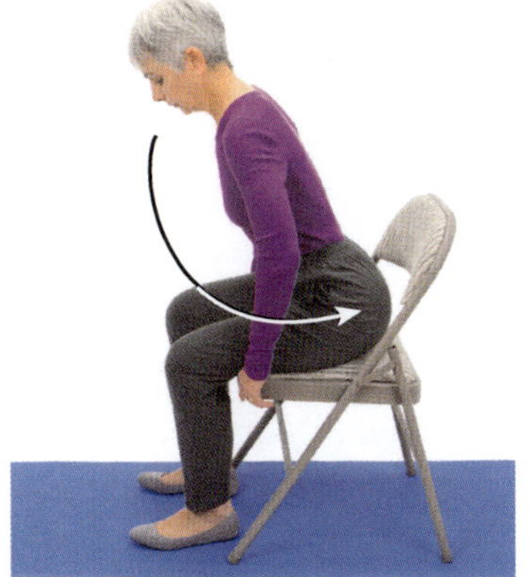

Figure 3

- Legs wide, squat down until your buttocks touch the chair seat *(figure 2)*.
- Lean forward and slide both buttocks in unison as far to the back of the seat as the comfort in your low back allows. Fig to make sure the weight is on your pubic bone *(figure 3)*.

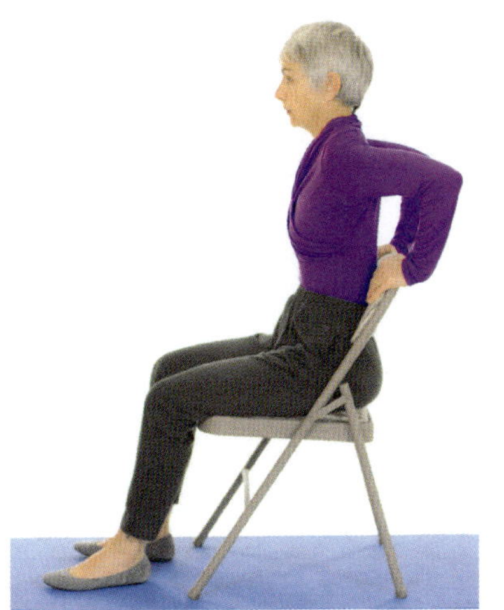

Figure 4

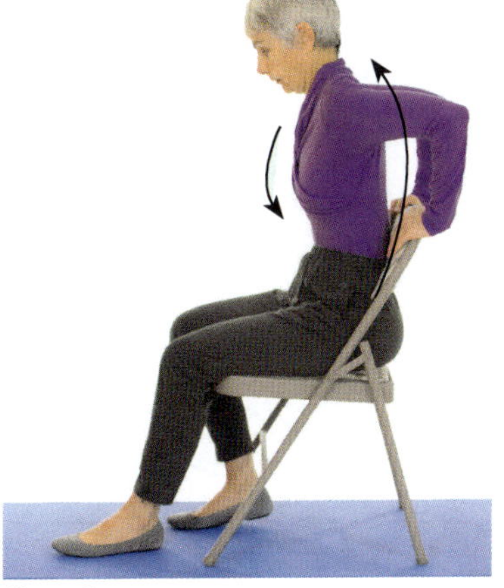

Figure 5

- Take hold of the sides of the chair back *(figure 4)*.
- Lengthen your lumbar spine: Lean forward and carefully fold down under your breasts. Keep your pelvis relaxed and heavy on the chair *(figure 5)*.

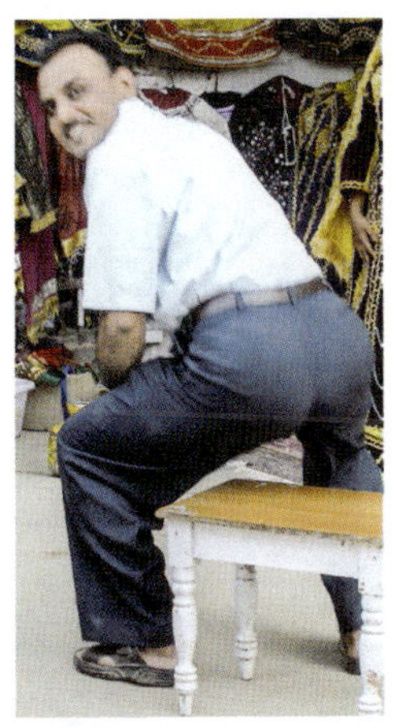

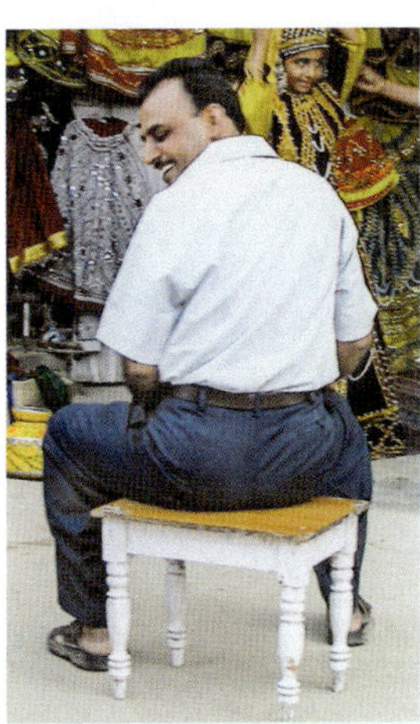

In Balance. Squatting to sit down: With legs wide, this man points his buttocks well behind him, then sits down.

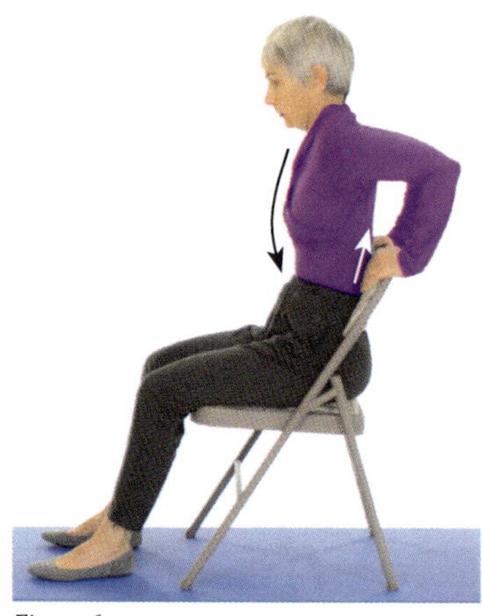
Figure 6

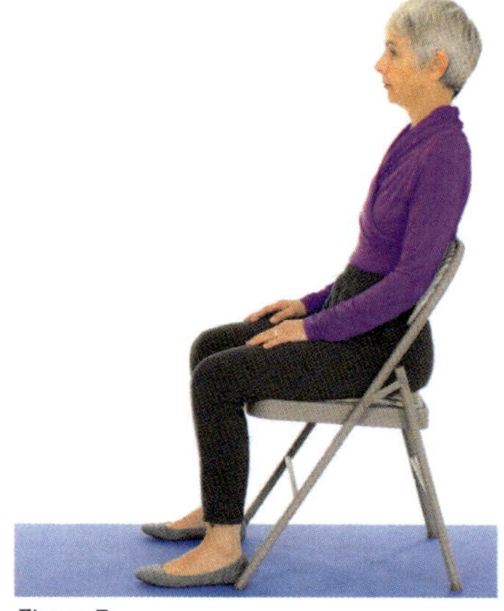
Figure 7

- Gently press down on your hands and feel your low back/lumbar area lift and lengthen. Hold this traction as you move back and rest against the chair *(figure 6)*.
- Press on your hands for a final lift, then let your hands rest on your thighs and relax. Your low back and belly will feel lifted as you relax against the chair *(figure 7)*.
- Drop your shoulders and let them be heavy. Bring your neck back and up, chin to throat, letting the back of the head rise from the hairline. Soften your jaw.
- Legs comfortably apart, feel weight in the front of your pelvis, close to your pubic bone, and let it settle there.
- Let your chest relax, ribs down. Rest lightly against the back of the chair.

RIBS DOWN

"Ribs down" is a reminder to drop the ribs. Never sit up straight by lifting the chest.

CHECK AND FEEL

☑ *How do you feel?*

Become conscious of any strain and let it go. Let your weight sink into the chair, especially in the front of the pelvis. Become aware of your breath and let it rise up your spine as you inhale. The more you relax, the more you will feel the breath like a massage.

☑ *Does the chair dig into your back?*

If your buttocks are too far back on the seat, the chair may dig uncomfortably into your back. Slide forward a little (both buttocks at the same time), lengthen your back again by pressing your hands down against the edge of the chair, lift and let go. Rest vertically, your back lightly against the chair and most of your weight on the seat, in the front of your pelvis.

☑ *Is your chin lifted?*

Lift your hair at the base of your skull. This will let the back of your neck rise and bring your chin down. It will also extend the top of your spine without strain.

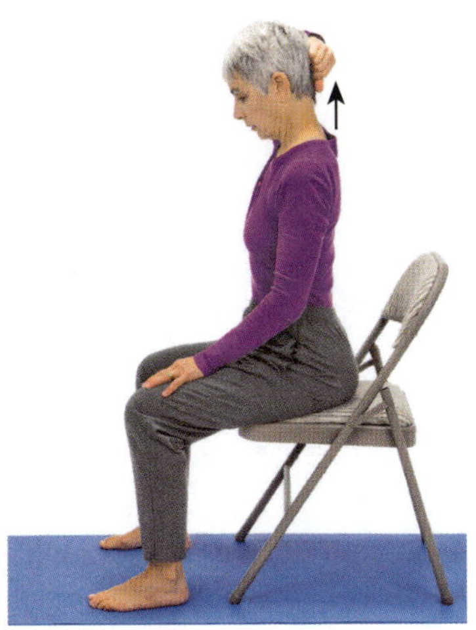

☑ *Is your upper back rounded?*

If your upper spine has a rounded shape it will straighten slowly over time as you change your habits. It all begins with learning how to sit with your weight in the front of the pelvis and straightening up from there. This elongation includes the head and neck. Carrying the head out in front of the body bends the spine unnaturally.

LUMBAR SUPPORT

Many people use lumbar support pillows, but remember that our goal is to flatten the lumbar curve and move it down to the natural arch. Placing a pillow at your lumbar spine will create a curve instead of length. If you need support, place a pillow behind your upper back, around the shoulder blades. Try this in an airplane seat and you will see how restful it is.

Aligning the Shoulders, Head, and Neck

Once you know how to sit comfortably, you will benefit from learning how to:

- Relax your shoulders
- Bring your head back and lengthen the neck

You will use these guidelines whether sitting or standing, but it is easiest to learn them while sitting.

In Balance. Notice how this woman's weight falls in front of her pelvis and her "behind" is well behind her. Her back, neck, and head form a straight line.

As you get used to sitting like this it becomes extremely comfortable and back support becomes optional.

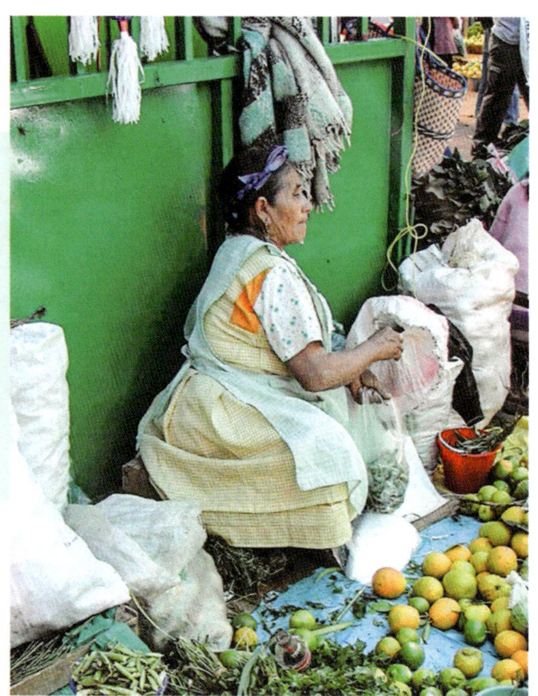

RELAXING YOUR SHOULDERS

When your pelvis and spine are in the right position, you will become more aware of the position of your shoulders. You may notice that they are forward or lifted or both—either one is a common cause of muscle tension.

To be in their natural position, your shoulders must be relaxed and pointing straight to the sides, shoulder blades flat on your back, and your upper arms hanging straight down at your sides. This position is possible only when you are aligned on the axis. It cannot be forced—you will only hurt yourself if you do shoulder exercises without first aligning your pelvis and spine.

To relieve shoulder tension it is necessary to become aware of your habits and let your shoulders settle, many times during the day. It is important to begin to *feel* the tension, to become aware of it until it "talks to you" and you are prompted to stop lifting your shoulders. This habit is hard to break!

A helpful practice for relaxing and placing your shoulders is the Shoulder Roll.

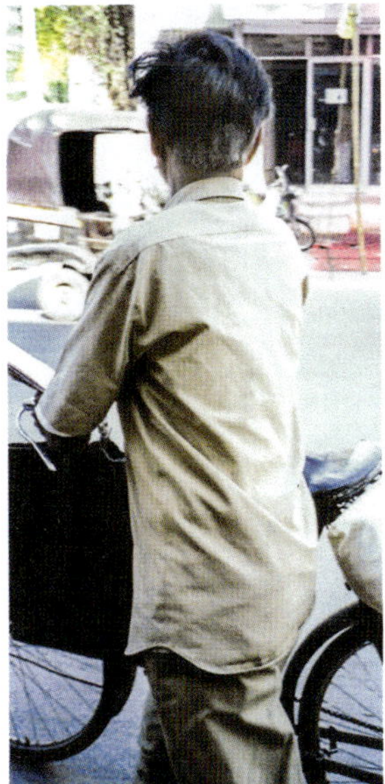

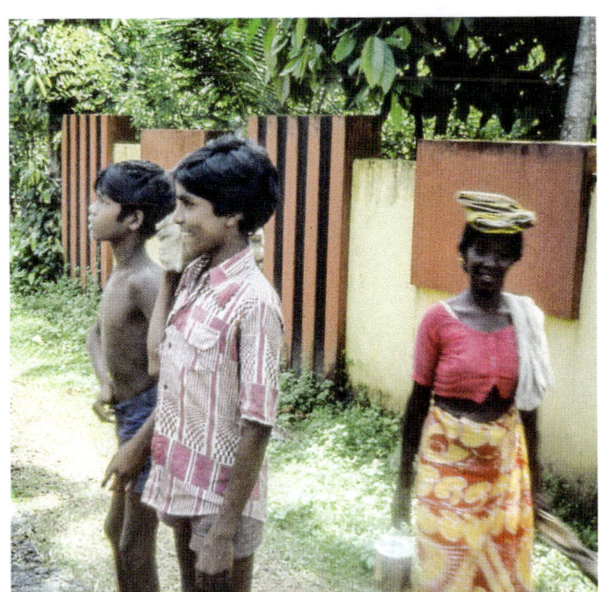

In Balance. (Left) The natural position of the shoulders is neither lifted nor forced back. The shoulder blades are flat. (Right) The chest is high and open with the shoulders pointing straight to the sides.

THE SHOULDER ROLL

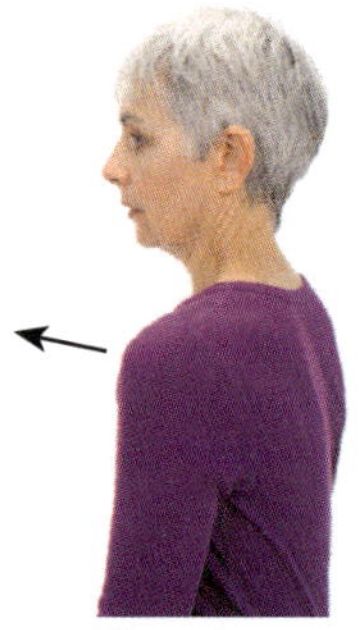

Figure 1

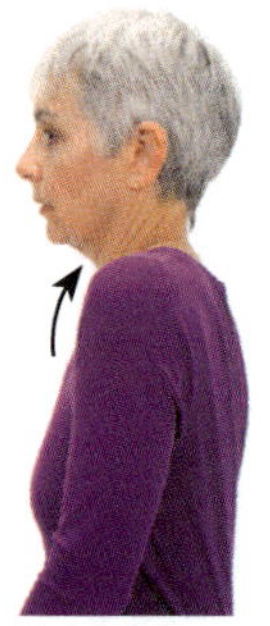

Figure 2

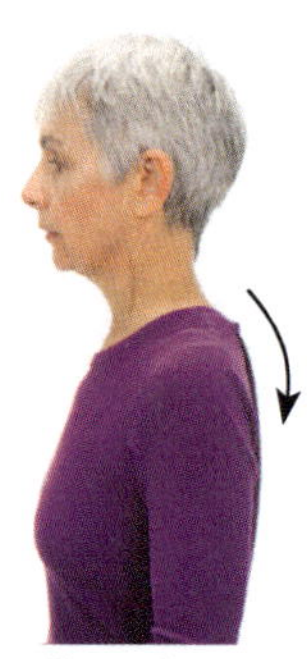

Figure 3

- Let your arms hang heavy by your side. Without moving any other part of your body, take one shoulder straight forward *(figure 1).*
- Lift it up, rotating toward your ear *(figure 2).*
- Lower it, moving your elbow back and away, and complete a circle by dropping the shoulder down *(figure 3).*
- Repeat with your other shoulder.

At first your shoulder may not be mobile enough to rotate smoothly in the socket. You may find that you move somewhere else to compensate. For example, you might lift your chest and arch your back. Concentrate on moving only at the shoulder socket and keep the spine undisturbed.

Repeat the Shoulder Roll several times during the day as a reminder to keep your shoulders dropped and back. Even just letting your shoulders hang heavy, arms straight down, will relax them.

BRINGING YOUR HEAD BACK

Centering the head on the trunk relieves strain on the neck and shoulders.

For many reasons, most people carry their head out in front of the trunk. This unnatural head position has become so common, especially among those who work at computers, that in medical circles it is called Forward Head Syndrome. Young children have not yet adopted this habit, and the difference between adults and children is often striking.

People who live in Balance have a straight neck centered on the trunk, not in front of it. Characteristic of this head position is a downward slope between the mid-ear and the bottom of the nose: The tip of the nose is always lower than the ear. The head rotates freely, without strain, because it is in line with the spine.

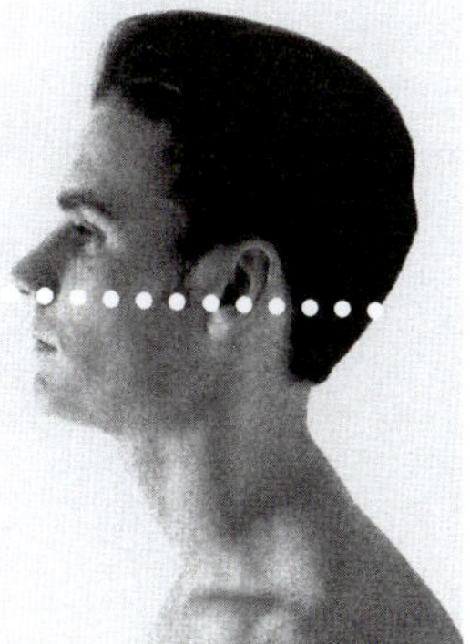

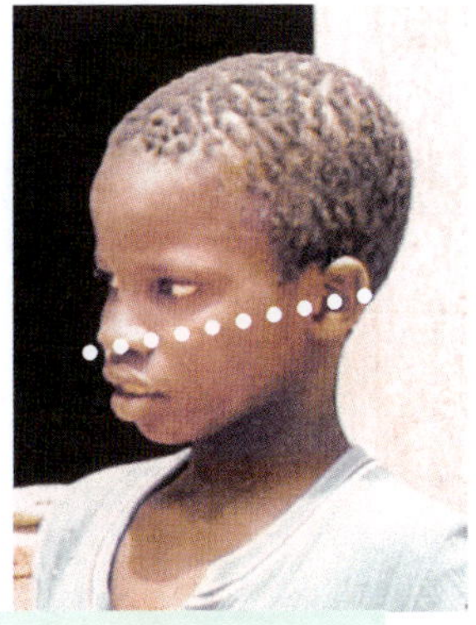

Notice the different head positions of the man and the boy.

Out of Balance. The man's chin is lifted and his head is forward relative to his trunk. **In Balance.** The boy has a long straight neck centered on his trunk and the tip of his nose is lower than the ear.

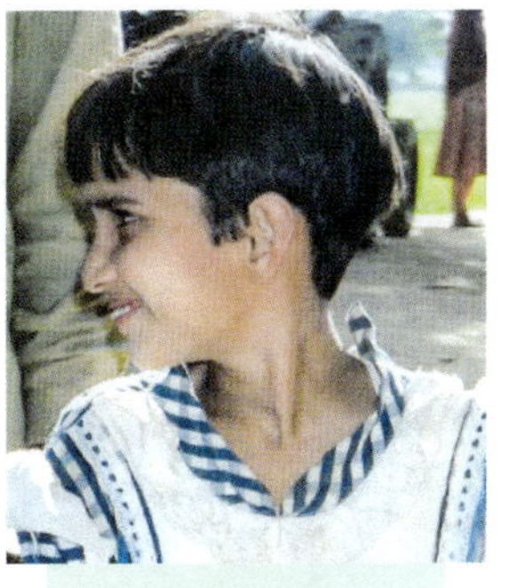

In Balance. When the neck is in line with the spine, the head can rotate freely on its axis.

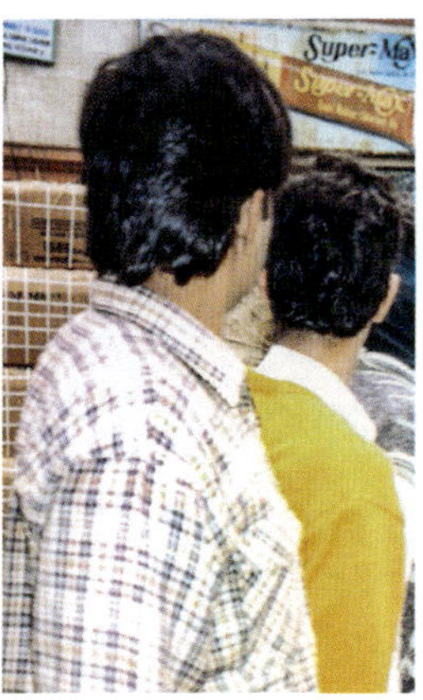

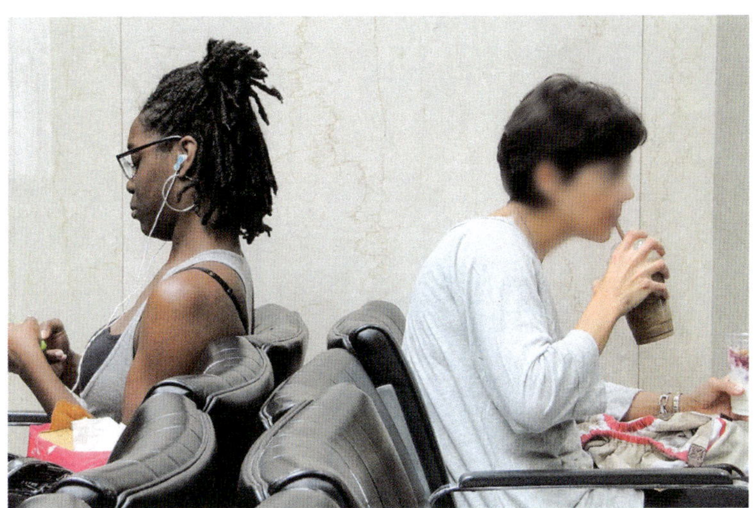

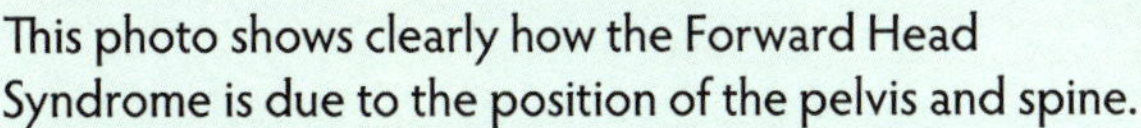

This photo shows clearly how the Forward Head Syndrome is due to the position of the pelvis and spine.

(Left) **In Balance.** This woman sits against the back of the chair with her whole spine, so her pelvis is well under her. Her spine follows a straight line into her neck.

(Right) **Out of Balance.** This woman sits on her tail-bone, forcing her spine into a semicircle. This brings her neck forward and arches the neck. As she gets older, pain will be inevitable.

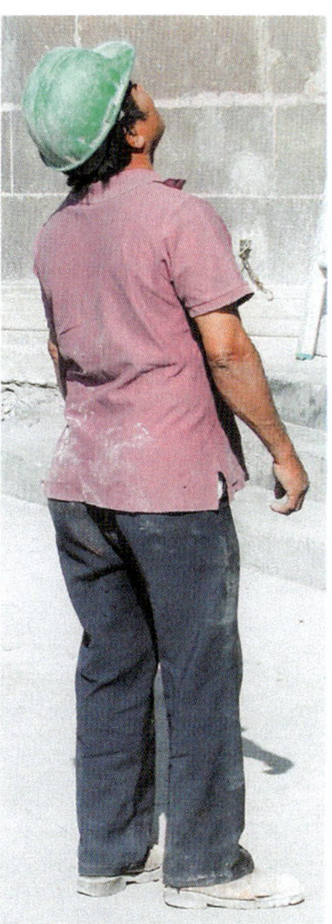

In Balance. The head is centered over the trunk. To look up, the head bends where the skull meets the neck, without arching the lower, middle part of the neck and squeezing the disks.

THE GOOSENECK STRETCH

To lengthen the neck and center the head on the trunk, it is helpful to do the Gooseneck Stretch.

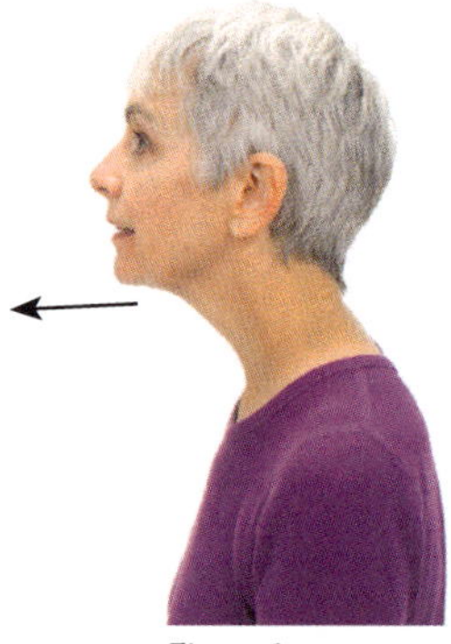

Figure 1

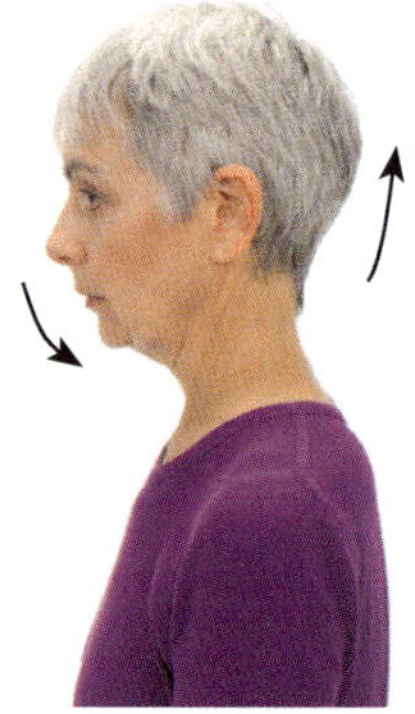

Figure 2

- Sit in Balance.
- Keeping your shoulders heavy, glide your chin forward from the base of your neck *(figure 1)*. Don't crease the back of your neck.
- Draw your chin in and bring your neck back and up, letting the back of the head rise from the hairline *(figure 2)*. Feel your head centered over your spine. Do not strain.
- Relax your jaw. Your face is vertical.

Repeat several times.

Sitting Without Back Support

When you sit with your weight on your pubic bone it is possible to sit very comfortably without back support. The spine can extend, which will relieve strain or pain in your low back. The corselet muscles are in a position to lengthen and support you naturally. You can sit at ease while working at your computer, playing the piano, eating, or doing any variety of daily activities.

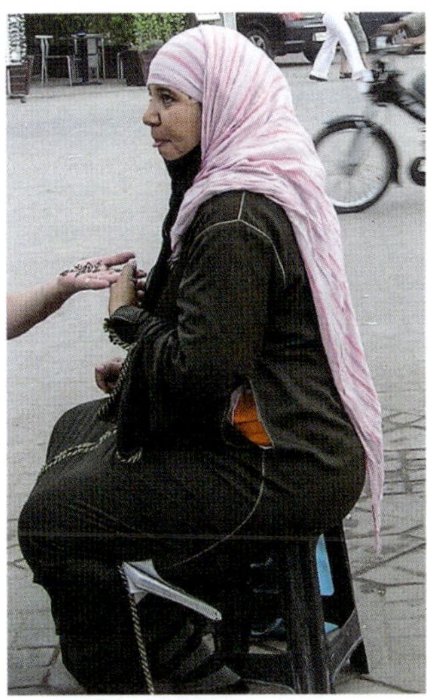

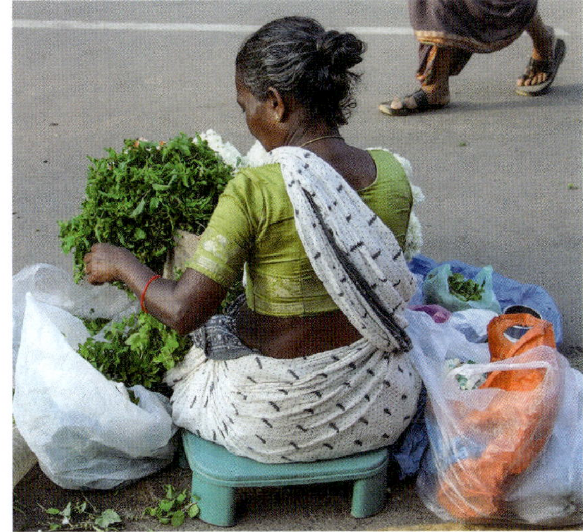

In Balance. (Left) Look closely and note that the Moroccan woman's weight rests on the front of her pelvis, on her pubic bone. Her legs slope down into a **V.** (Right) Sitting on a low stool, the same principles apply.

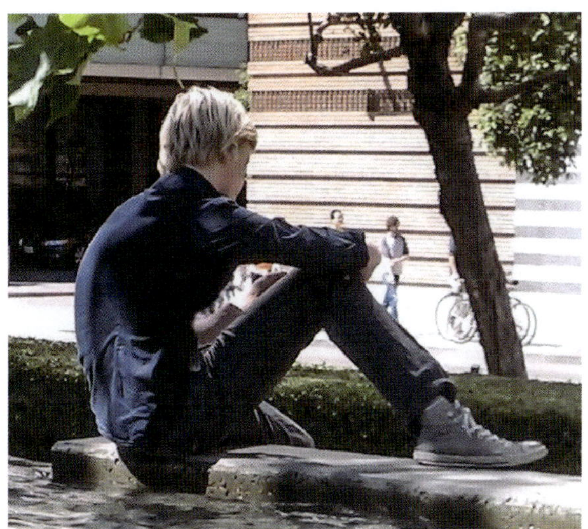

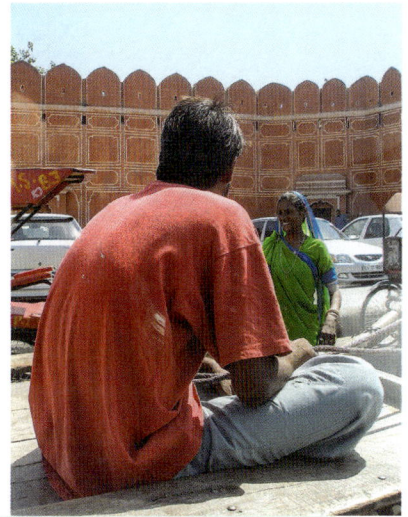

Out of Balance. In contrast, these young men sit on their tailbone, with the pelvis hiked up in front. They have to round the back and arch the neck to look straight ahead. Both men are likely to experience back pain and look stooped and old at an early age.

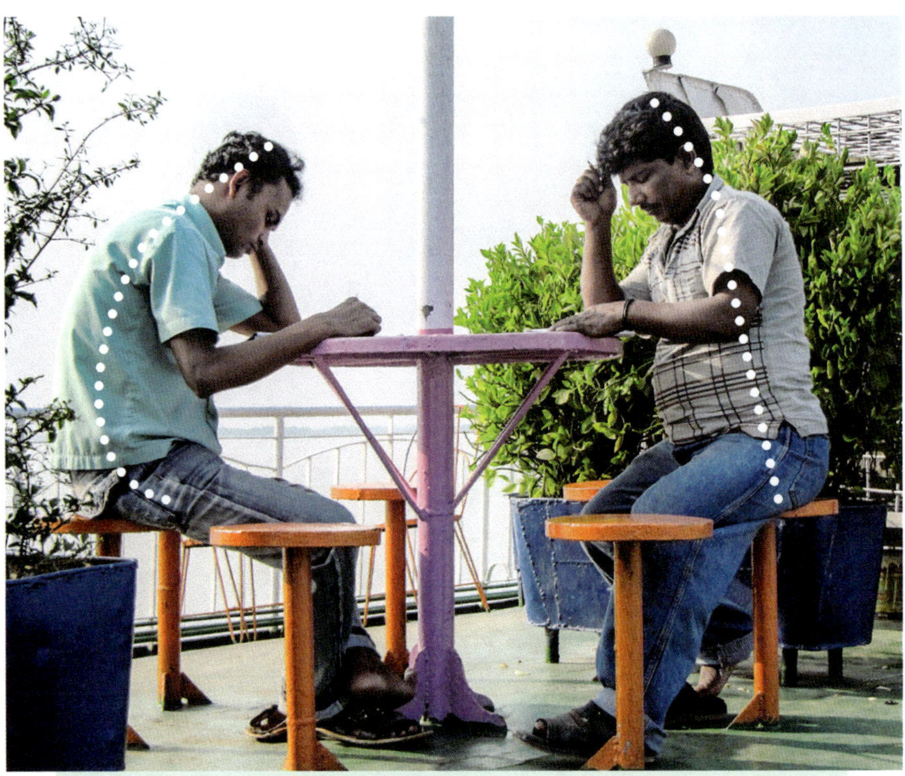

Notice the chain reaction in both bodies, beginning with the position of the pelvis.

(Left) **Out of Balance**. The pelvis is collapsed backward (pubic bone is lifted), the natural arch is rounded, and the thoracic spine is rounded. The weight of the forward head pulls the neck, upper back, and shoulders forward. The head is lifted to counter this forward line, arching the neck (chin forward).

(Right) **In Balance.** The pelvis is forward (weight is in front, at the pubic bone), the spine is extended from the natural arch, and the head is close to the body. The head is bent at the base of the skull (chin tucked). The right arm rests lightly on the table. Shoulders are down.

HOW TO PRACTICE

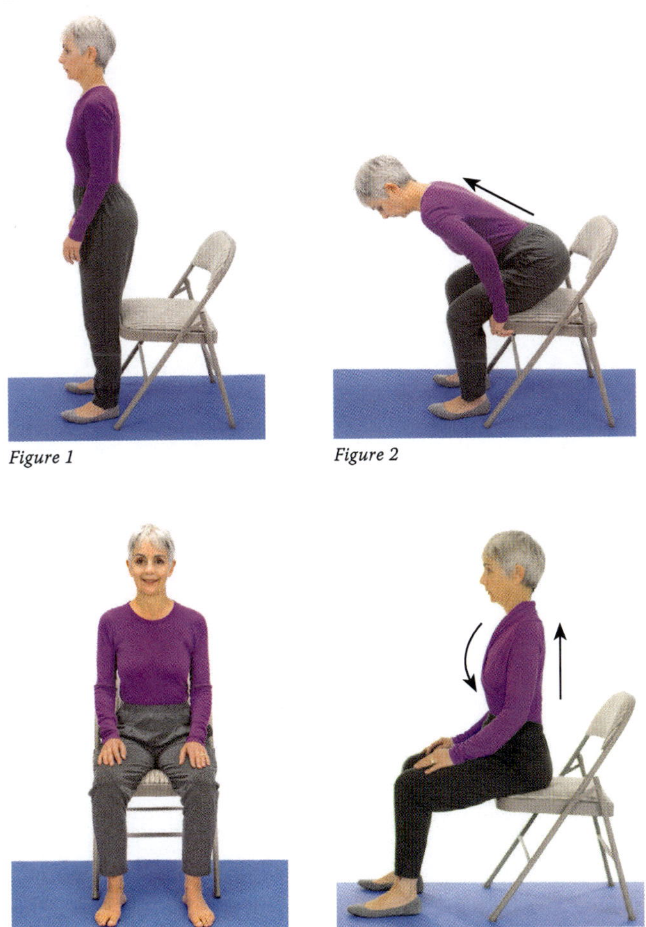
Figure 1 *Figure 2*
Figure 3 *Figure 4*

- Stand close to the seat of the chair *(figure 1).*
- Squat until your buttocks touch the seat, and sit down *(figure 2).*
- Legs comfortably apart, feel weight in the front of your pelvis, close to your pubic bone, and fig to let it settle there *(figure 3).*
- Let your chest relax, ribs down. Follow the line *(figure 4).*
- Do a Shoulder Roll: One at a time, bring your shoulders forward, up, back, and down. (See The Shoulder Roll on page 46.)
- Bring your neck back and up, letting the back of the head rise from the hairline. Feel your head centered over your spine.
- Place your heels directly under your knees.
- Feel your breath lift and expand the top of your chest.

CHECK AND FEEL

☑ *Where do you feel weight?*

When you begin practicing this, you will feel your sitting bones under you, which means that they are bearing your weight. Gradually you will be able to relax more and increase the forward rotation of the pelvis until you feel weight in the pubic bone. This takes time to learn. It requires more and more letting go. It cannot be forced.

☑ *Does your low back feel tense?*

"Re-fig": With both hands on the chair seat between your legs, lean forward and lift your buttocks. Aim your fig leaf farther back and down between your legs, and sit down *(figure 1)*. Use a wedge or small cushion under your sitting bones to help train the pelvis to relax in this position *(figure 2)*.

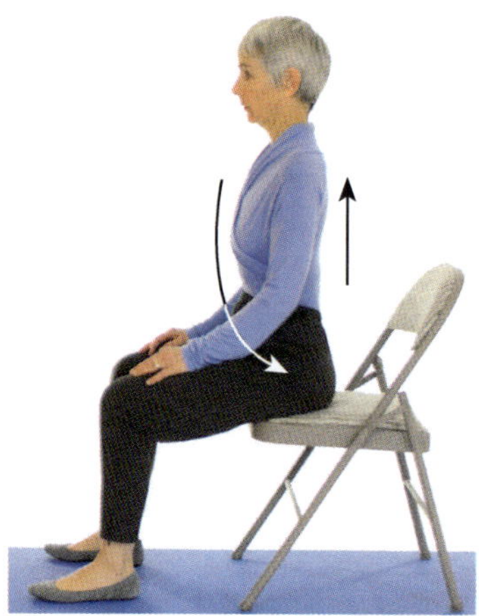

Figure 1

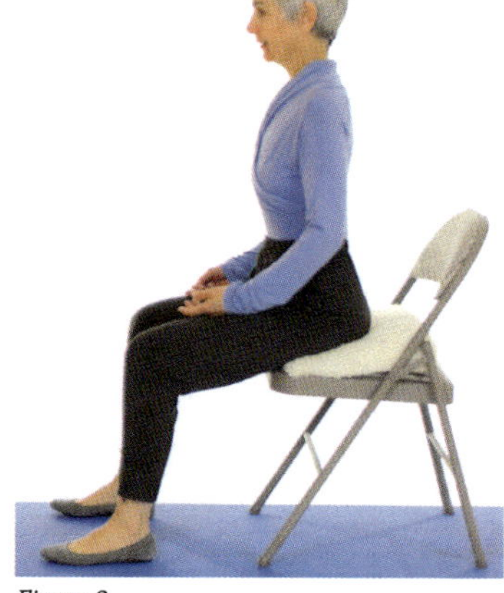

Figure 2

☑ *Are your shoulders tense?*

Lifting your shoulders causes tension. Often this is a long-held habit and feels normal until it begins to hurt. Each time the tension becomes apparent, neutralize it by lifting and dropping your shoulders several times. Bring your neck back and up, and relax your jaw.

Repeat the Shoulder Roll and Gooseneck Stretch several times during the day. (See the Shoulder Roll on page 46 and the Gooseneck Stretch on page 48.)

☑ *Are your knees higher than your hips?*

The chair is too low. Elevate the seat with a firm wedge (a pillow or folded blanket) if a higher seat is not available. You will be more comfortable if your thighs slope down slightly toward your knees.

☑ *Do you feel even pressure on both sitting bones?*

Only when your weight is evenly distributed will you feel exactly the same on the left and right sides of your pelvis. It takes practice to notice this imbalance because you are so used to it. But an uneven pelvis will cause uneven wear on hips and vertebrae, inviting injury.

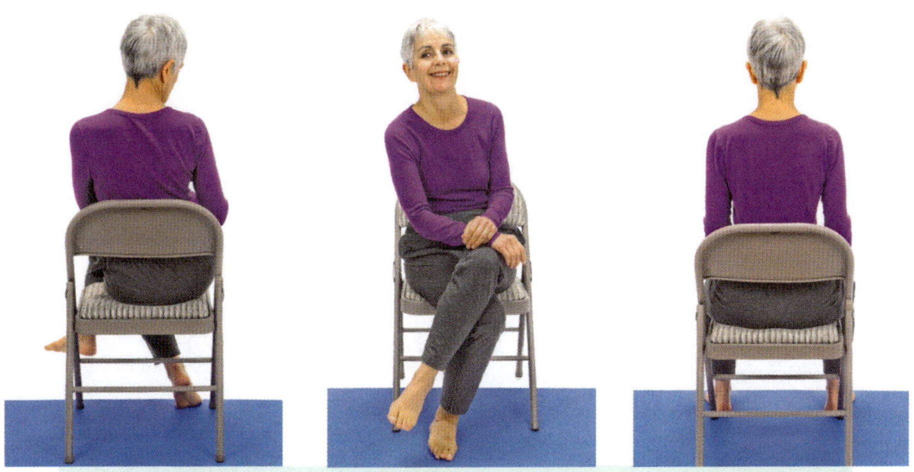

(Left and center) **Out of Balance.** Crossed knees, leaning to one side, a collapsed chest, and a lifted chin are common habits to be unlearned. All these place your pelvis unevenly. (Right) **In Balance.** A healthy habit is to sit down as if in a squat, which centers your pelvis and seats you solidly and upright.

Getting Up from a Chair

A common way to get up from a chair is to place the hands on the thighs, or other surface, and push up from there. You can imagine how this wears on the shoulders, since they do the lifting. Getting up from a chair in Balance shifts the work to the large bones in the lower part of your body. If the pelvis pivots at the hips and the legs do the lifting, your shoulders will thank you. With practice, getting up from a chair will feel easier and look more graceful.

HOW TO PRACTICE

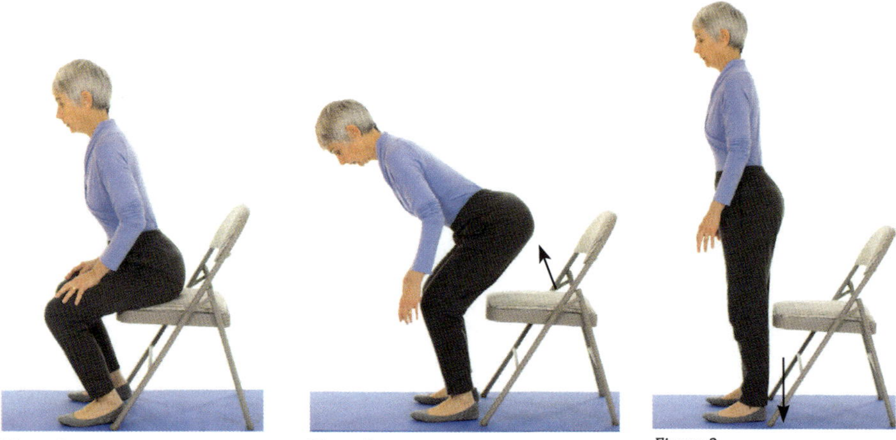

Figure 1 *Figure 2* *Figure 3*

- Slide to the front edge of your seat. Place your feet just under your chair, knees wide. Keep them wide, heels slightly lifted *(figure 1).*
- Rock forward until the weight of your torso lifts your buttocks off the chair and your body hovers over your feet *(figure 2).*
- In a continuing movement, simply straighten your legs, keeping weight in your heels *(figure 3).*

CHECK AND FEEL

☑ *Not so easy?*

Be sure to start from the edge of your seat. Move your feet farther under your chair.

☑ *Do you still feel too much effort?*

You are forcing somewhere. You imagine that you have to do too much.

It is helpful to think of balancing weight and counterweight, as on a seesaw. In this case your upper body is one weight, your pelvis another. When the trunk moves forward, the pelvis lifts by itself.

Reclining on a Chair

Reclining differs from sitting with back support in that it implies a leaning back against the support of a chair or couch to relax.

When you recline, the shape of the chair (its height and depth) is not so critical as when you sit upright. As for the height, let your legs slope down by stretching them out in front, crossed at the ankles or not. As for the depth, you will probably find it easier in the beginning to recline on a straight-backed chair with a seat that is not deeper than the length of your thighs. This will make it easier to keep your weight in front.

A deep chair or couch will require a firm pillow to fill in the gap between your back and the seat back. If you have to lean back too far, your pelvis will hike up in front and you will sit on your tailbone. Either shorten the seat by placing a firm pillow against the seat back, or lean against a pillow that is placed behind your upper back—at and just below the shoulder blades.

Compare the photos below. When a person sits in Balance the pelvis angles down in front and the spine does not round.

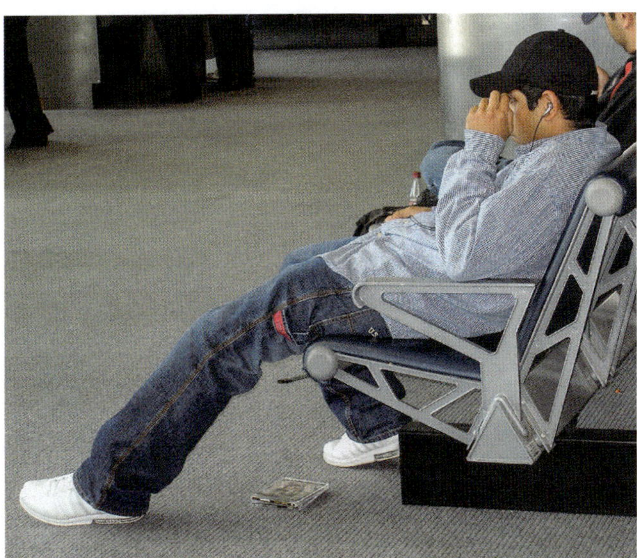

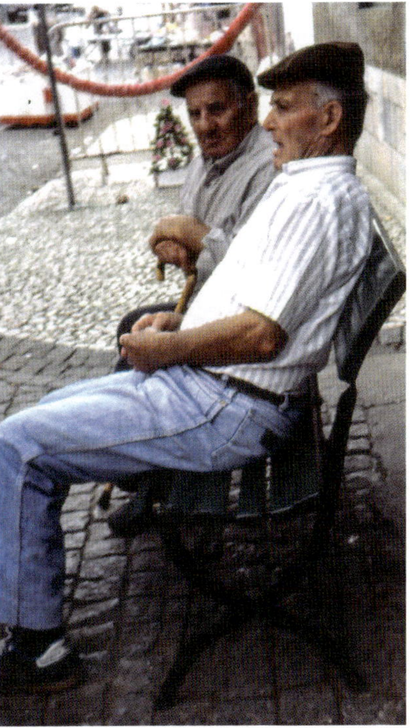

Out of Balance. If you are used to sitting like the man above, it is harmful and after a while you will need to shift and change position.

In Balance. The man at right can sit comfortably for long periods, perfectly still.

HOW TO PRACTICE

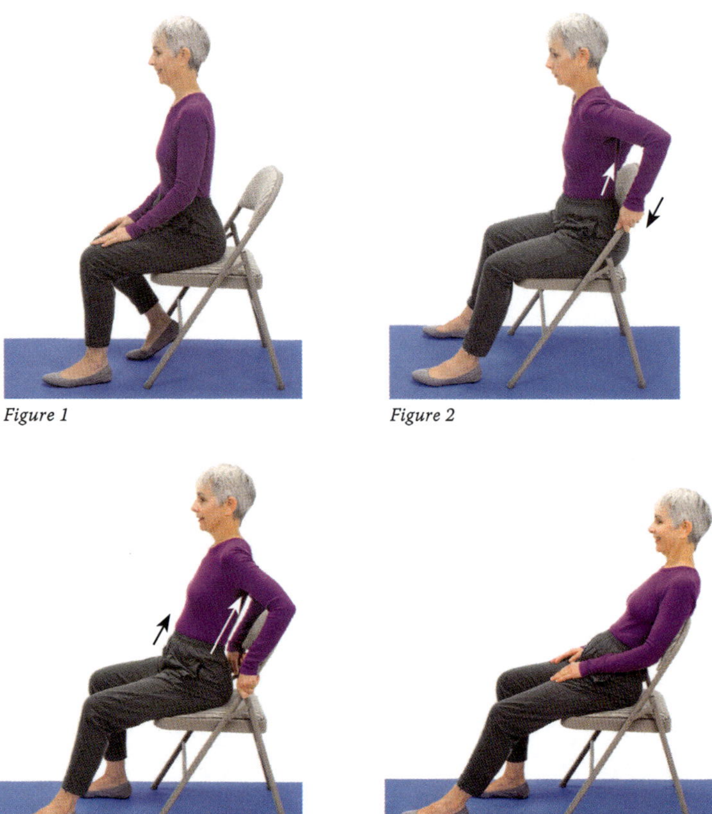

Figure 1 *Figure 2* *Figure 3* *Figure 4*

- Sit in Balance midseat on a chair, and fig so your weight is in the front of your pelvis (on your pubic bone) *(figure 1)*.
- Press down with your hands on the side edge of the seat, lean forward, and lengthen your back with the downward pressure of your hands *(figure 2)*.
- Hold this lift in your back and belly as you lean back against the chair. Feel length in your low back and abdomen *(figure 3)*.
- Relax your shoulders and let them settle *(figure 4)*.
- Bring your neck back and up, letting the back of the head rise from the hairline.
- Stretch your legs out in front, perhaps crossing them at your ankles.
- Relax everywhere. Feel weight in the front of your pelvis.

CHECK AND FEEL

☑ *Do you feel comfortable?*

Relax everywhere and let the chair carry your weight.

If you feel too far forward and are leaning back too much, reduce the angle. Slide a couple of inches farther back on your chair, fig, and try again until it feels very comfortable.

☑ *You don't feel your sitting bones?*

To feel your sitting bones, you need the fig leaf to stay down between your legs. This happens by itself if your weight stays in the front of your pelvis as you lean back. Keep your chest weighted down in front. Your pubic bone anchors you as you lean back.

Try again: Fig, lift, lean back, let go.

☑ *You don't feel length in your back and belly?*

The chest (ribs) may have lifted as you leaned back. Try again: Anchor your pubic bone and, as you lean back, keep your ribs heavy. Now feel both the front (abdomen) and back of your trunk participate in the stretch.

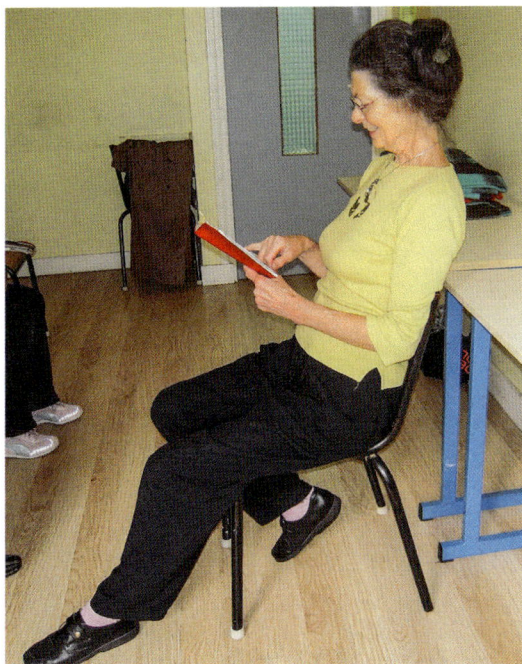

In Balance. Georgia, a teacher at the Aplomb Institute, reclines on a straight-backed chair with the pelvis angled down in front, allowing her spine to lengthen. She sits relaxed and comfortable. Notice the casual position of her legs.

Farmer's Rest

People all over the world are able to sit and rest comfortably in a foward-leaning position. We call this the Farmer's Rest because of its traditional image.

Out of Balance. In Western culture it is common to see the positions shown here: rounded back, forward head, and sitting on the back of the pelvis.

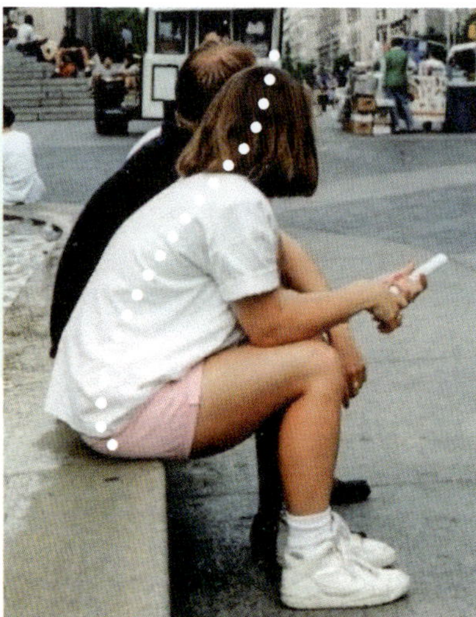

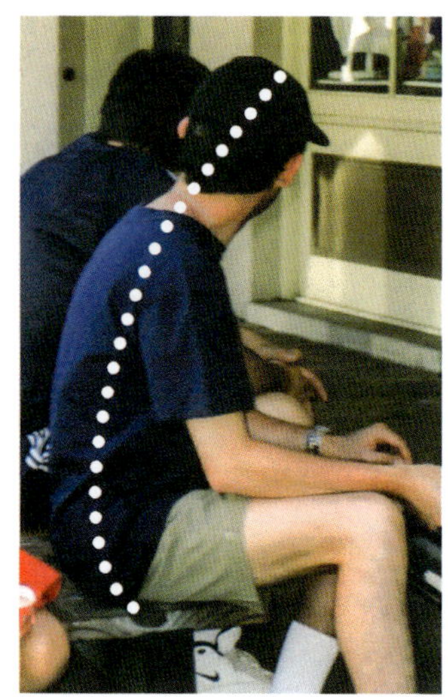

In Balance. The Bhutanese woman, in contrast, rests her weight on the front of her pelvis, bending at the hips with a straight spine. Her arms rest lightly on her thighs.

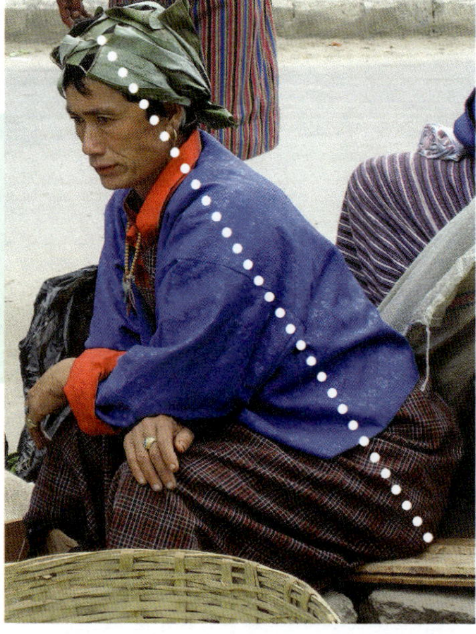

HOW TO PRACTICE

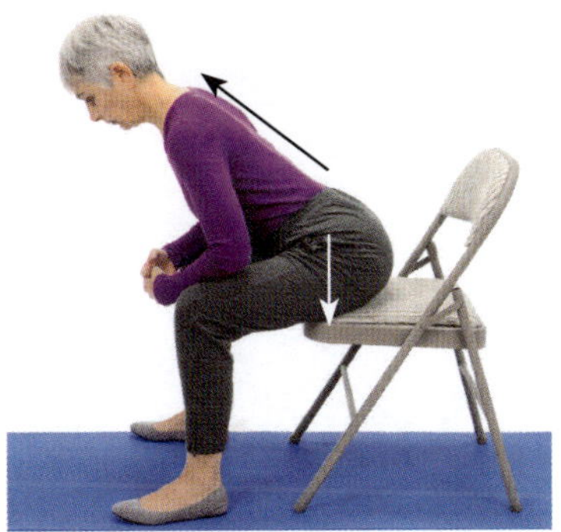

- Sit midseat on a chair or bench, and fig.
- Press your hands down on your thighs, lengthen your spine up from your hip joints and, holding this lift, bend forward at your hips with a straight spine.
- Let your arms rest lightly on your thighs, just above your knees. Feel weight on the chair as if you were sitting on your pubic bone. Let your weight settle there, and release it.
- Relax your back. Feel the breath there.
- Bring your neck back and up, letting the back of the head rise from the hairline.
- Place your heels directly under your knees.
- Relax everywhere.

CHECK AND FEEL

☑ *Do you feel tension in your shoulders?*

Farmer's Rest is not easy at first, although it looks like it should be. The secret again is the position of the pelvis: The weight needs to be in the front, at your pubic bone. Then relax the whole pelvis and deliberately release your weight onto the chair.

Fig again, folding deeper at your hips into a squat. Bend forward at the hips and rest your arms lightly on your thighs. Take time to really feel most of your weight on the chair. Then the shoulders can relax. Don't worry about holding your pelvis in the right place; just let it have weight.

Sitting in a Car to Drive

This is similar to sitting with back support, but adjusted to the shape of a car.

- Stand next to the car seat and turn so that your back is toward the seat. Sit on the outside edge of the seat. Then bring one foot at a time into the car as you swivel around to face the front.
- Slide both buttocks to the back of the seat and fig.
- Most likely you are now sitting farther back in the seat than usual, so adjust the seat as needed to reach the pedals.
- Lean forward a little, press your hands down on the seat, and lengthen your low back. Hold this traction as you lean back against the seat.
- Bring your neck back and up, letting the back of the head rise from the hairline, and relax your jaw. Your face is vertical. Adjust the mirrors as needed.
- Drop your shoulders and let them be heavy.
- Hold the sides of the steering wheel gently—hands relaxed, palms in, thumbs up.

(Left) **Out of Balance.** Jean Couch sits well back on the seat, but the shape of the seat creates a curved spine and the headrest forces her head forward. She looks slumped.

(Right) **In Balance.** She placed a small wedge under her hips and a pillow behind her upper back to fill in the hollow back of the car seat. Notice the forward tilt of her pelvis. Her back is straight and she looks taller.

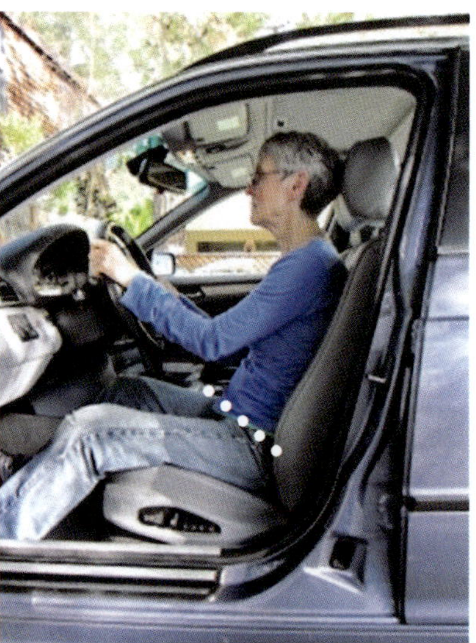

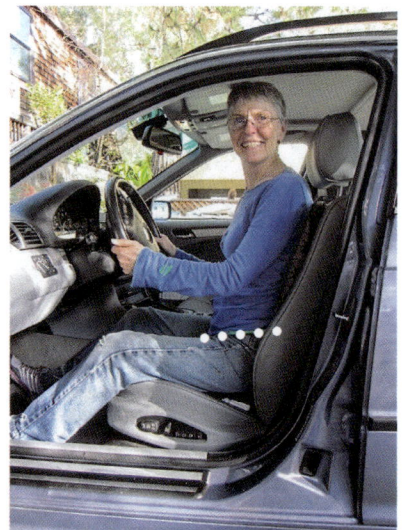

CHECK AND FEEL

☑ *Does your back feel arched?*

Car seats vary but are often quite curved, forcing your upper back to round. Experiment with a small pillow at your upper back to fill in the hollow seat, as shown in the photo on the previous page.

If the seat is slippery, cover the back with a yoga mat strip or nonslip fabric, like the kind used to prevent throw rugs from sliding.

Adjust the seat to a vertical position so that you don't have to lean back too far.

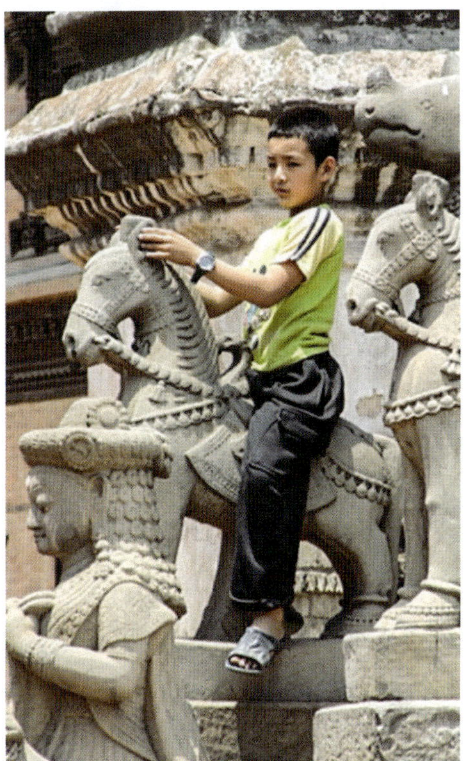

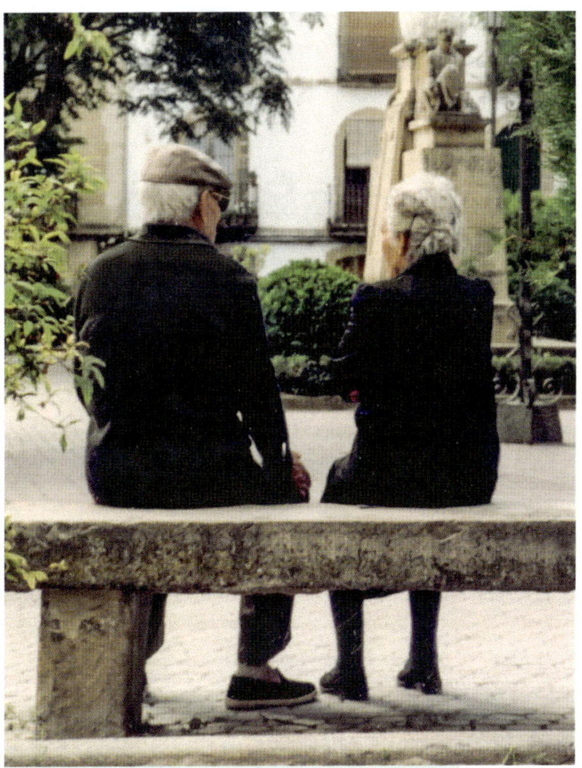

In Balance. The art of sitting can be practiced at any age. Look at the relaxed pelvis of the young boy and his long spine that seems to reach up. The elderly couple in a Spanish village sat comfortably on a concrete bench for a long time without moving in the slightest.

Using the Breath as a Guide When Sitting

When you are on the axis, the breath naturally massages your spine. You can feel this when sitting quietly.

- Take some time to sit well, with your weight in the front of your sitting bones. Lengthen your spine by engaging the corselet and following the line up from your natural arch. It is helpful to focus more on the back than the front.

- Relax your shoulders and focus on your breath. With practice you will feel the movement of your breath all the way up your spine, even up to a slight nodding of your head. If you feel no movement with the breath, there is tension or misalignment inhibiting this gentle undulation.

Normal breathing employs the intercostal muscles between your ribs, a crosshatch of muscles that allows for expansion (upward movement) and contraction (downward movement) of the rib cage. Only when your spine is on the axis is this up and down movement clearly felt all the way up to the base of your neck. This is a helpful checkpoint if you wonder, Am I doing it right?

Guiding the breath toward an area of tension will increase sensation and gradually bring release. Breathing with awareness invites tranquility in body and mind. The power of the breath is not to be underestimated!

THE BREATH AS A PUMP

As you breathe, the up and down movement of the ribs massages your spine and functions as a pump to circulate spinal fluid. Your ribs connect in front to the breastbone (sternum) and in back to the spine, where each rib is inserted between two vertebrae.

When your spine is aligned along the axis, the tip of each rib—where it inserts into the spine—operates like the tip of a screwdriver. It moves up and down with the breath and separates the vertebrae a tiny bit with each movement.

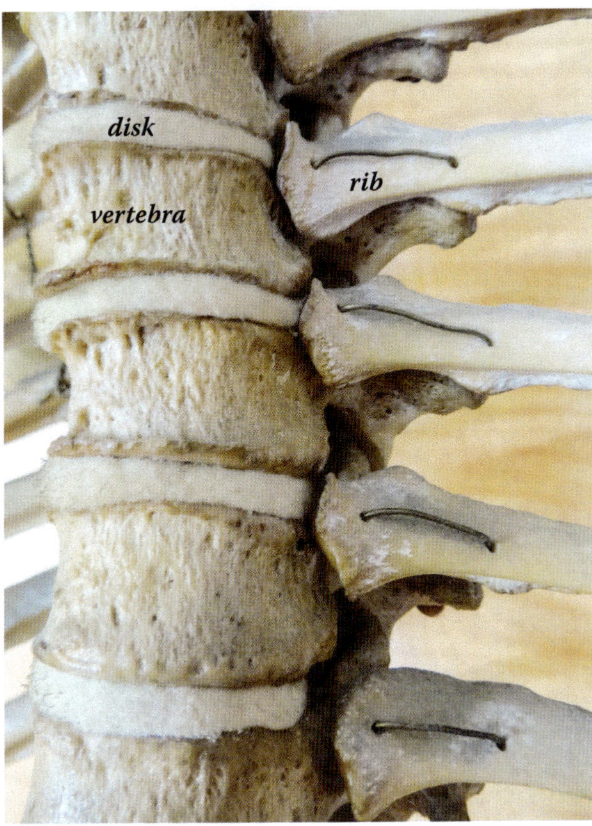

A section of the spine: The ribs attach between the vertebrae. The up and down movement of the ribs gently massages the spine.

STANDING IN BALANCE

> *If you will stand in the manner usually taught, back rigidly erect, knees, hips, and neck firm, chest held high, shoulders squared, head up and chin in, with abdomen retracted, then try to jump, you will find that you must* relax from *this strained attitude before you can make a move! This will serve to illustrate why the Indians consider the white man's posture ridiculous. Indians tell me that they cannot bear to have their children taught such an absurd posture in their schools, it is so strained, awkward and useless.*
>
> ~ Maud Smith Williams [16]

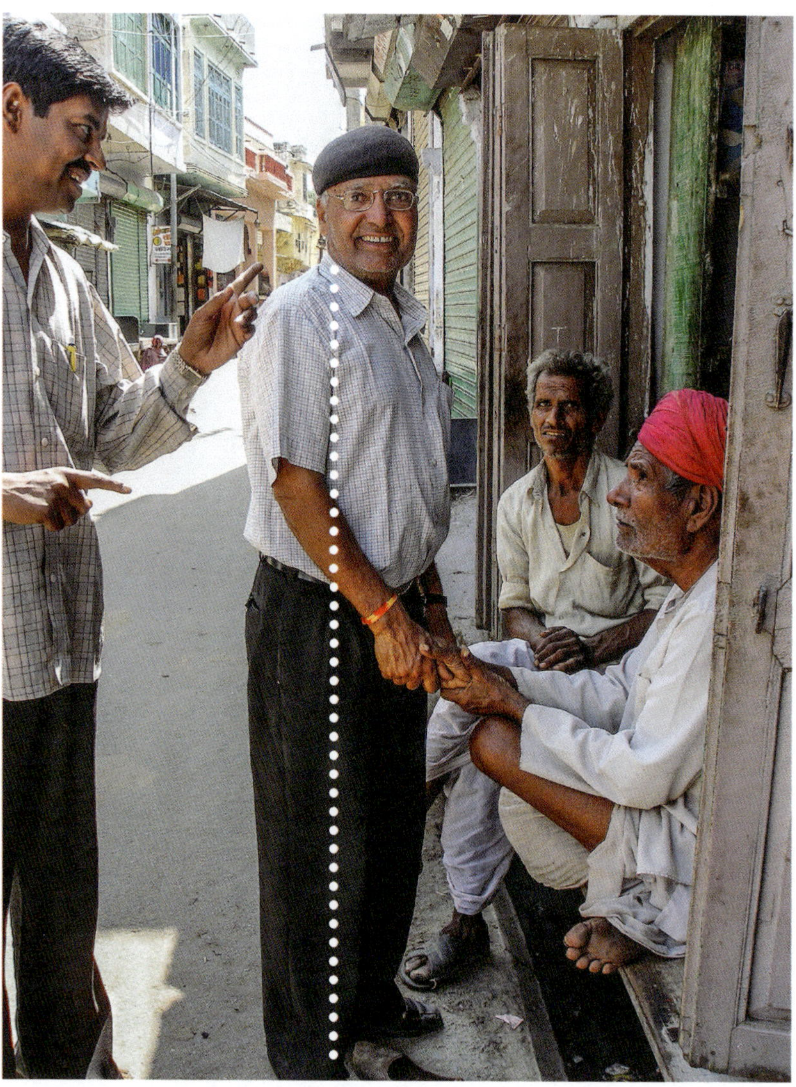

Standing with grace and without tension, naturally upright.

Standing with Ease

To stand gracefully and with ease, your spine must follow the axis of gravity (the plumb line). It requires your support bones—spine, pelvis, legs—to be stacked vertically.

When this is not the case, your muscles and tendons instead of the bones do most of the work of holding you up. This is inefficient and harmful. It creates muscle and joint tension, instability, and fatigue—and can lead to chronic pain.

The secret to standing is to place your weight so your bones can fully support you. It does not matter how heavy, large, or even overweight you are—you can still stand in Balance.

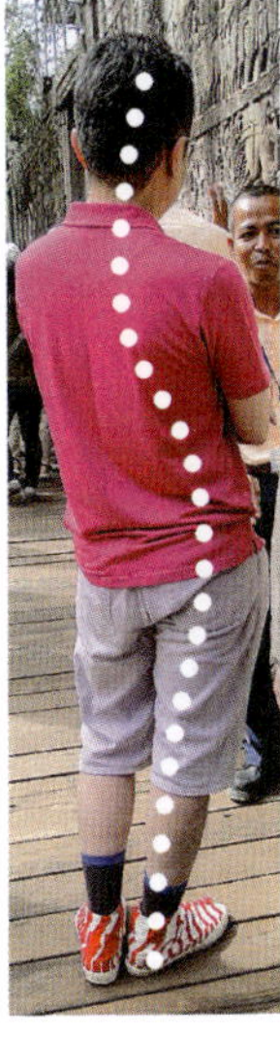

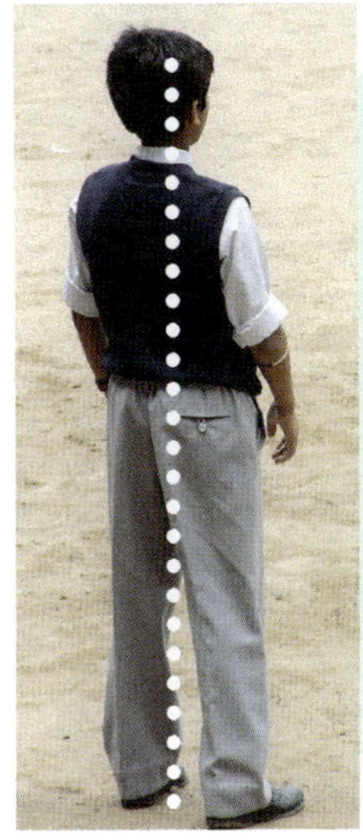

BACK VIEW
(Left) **Out of Balance.** The man's pelvis is pushed forward, the spine is in a zigzag shape, and the hips lean to one side. There are no visible, shaped buttocks.

(Right) **In Balance.** The pelvis (pubic bone) is down in front and the spine extends upward in a straight line. The buttocks are strong and muscular.

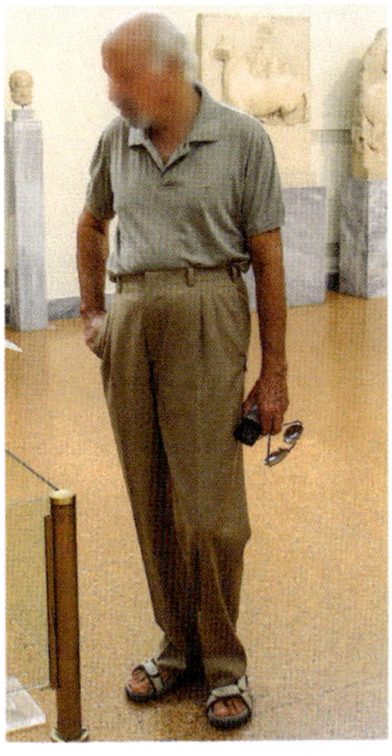

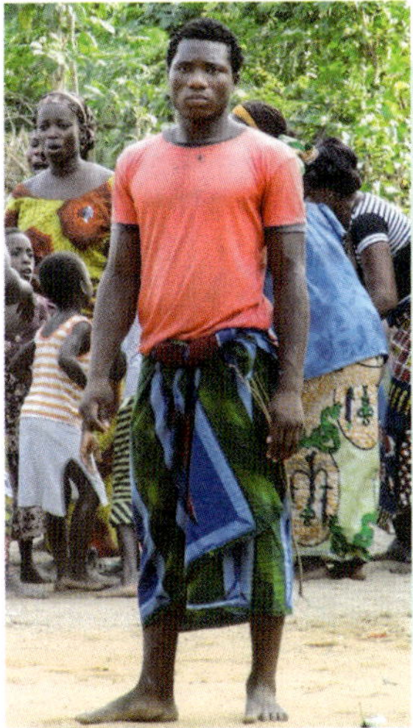

FRONT VIEW
(Left) **Out of Balance.** The pelvis is pushed forward, so the spine must round and the head and neck come forward.

(Right) **In Balance.** The pelvis (pubic bone) drops down in front and the spine extends upward into the neck. The head is centered on the trunk.

SIDE VIEW

In Balance. (Left) Notice the boy's alignment: You can draw a straight line from his head to his center hip and heel. (Right) Notice this boy's strong high buttock muscles, well-formed natural arch, long spine, and straight neck.

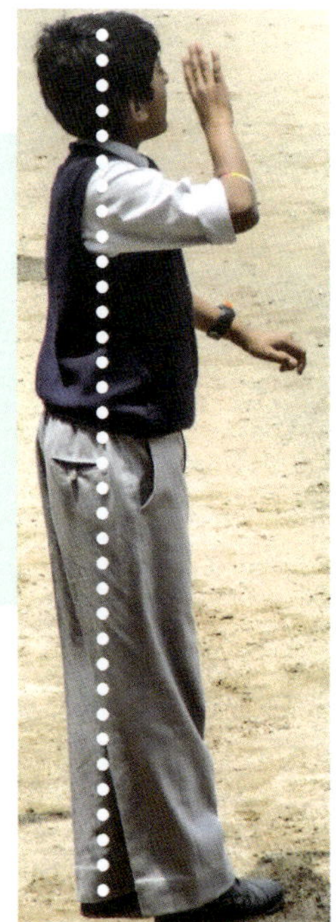

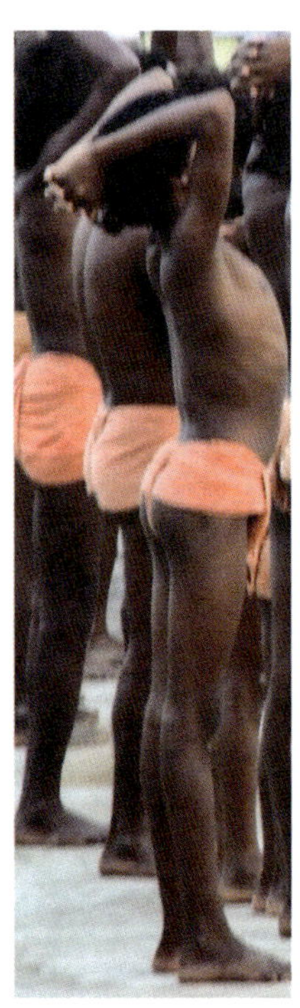

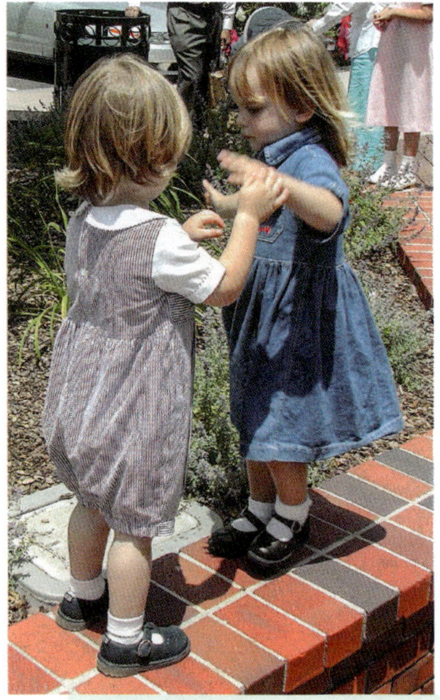

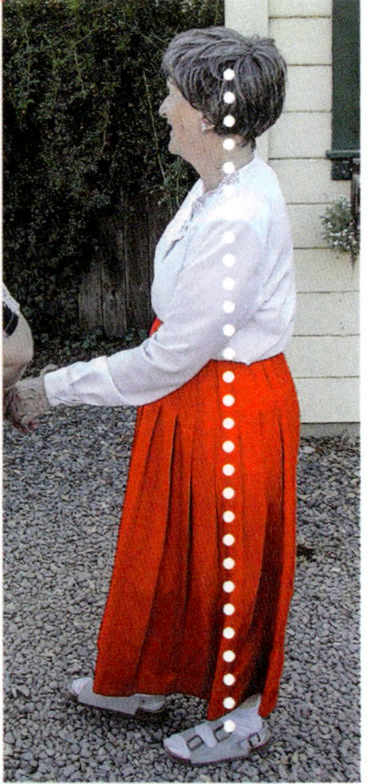

In Balance. Young children are perfectly aligned. The woman is 90 years old and stands the same way she did as a young girl.

HOW TO PRACTICE

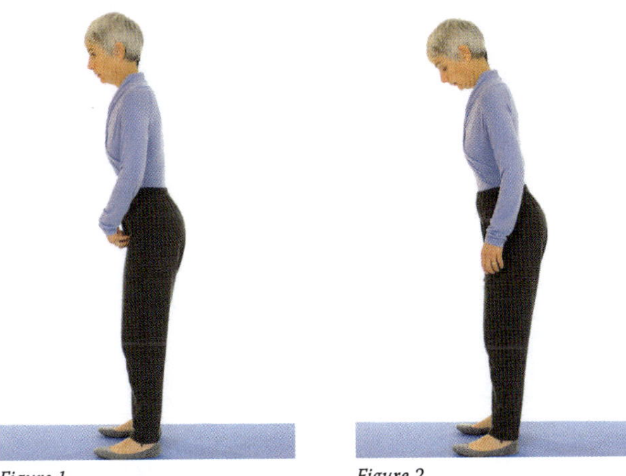

Figure 1 *Figure 2*

- Stand with your feet hip-width apart and in a slight **V,** with your legs on the median line (hips over knees over second toe).
- Locate your hip sockets: Touch the crease where your leg meets your trunk; in the center is your hip socket *(figure 1).*
- Bend slightly from that point and look at your ankles *(figure 2).* This takes weight into your heels.

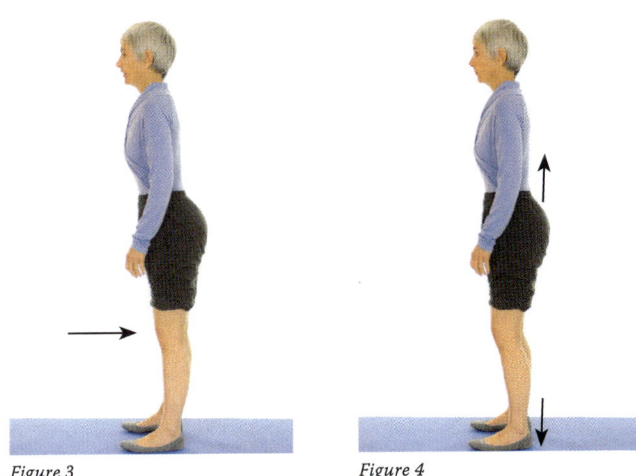

Figure 3 *Figure 4*

- If your knees are locked *(as in figure 3),* bend them a little. You will feel slightly seated, but more upright, and with weight in your heels.
- Straighten up from your natural arch, pressing down slightly on the heels and stretching up front and back without lifting your ribs or arching your back. Concentrate on your back and your front will follow *(figure 4).*

LOOK AT YOUR ANKLES

"Look at your ankles" is a reminder to rotate your pelvis forward and down until you feel weight in your heels. Let the tops of your legs move back far enough to see your ankles. Leave the pelvis in that position.

- Reach around and feel your lumbar spine. If it is hollow, drop your ribs and feel the spine relax. Then repeat stretching up from the natural arch. The ribs stay down.

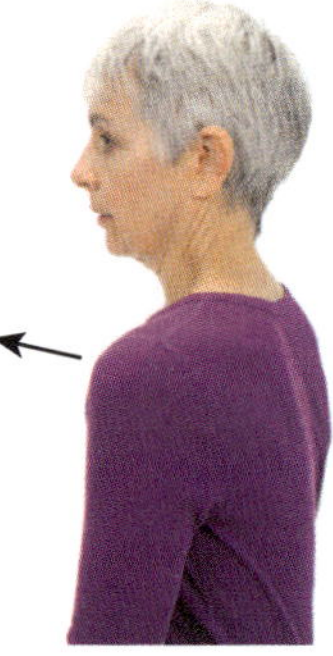

Figure 5

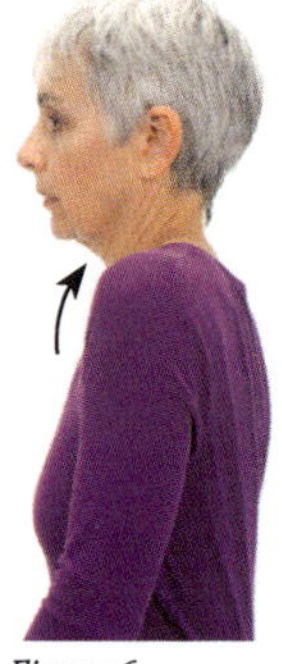

Figure 6

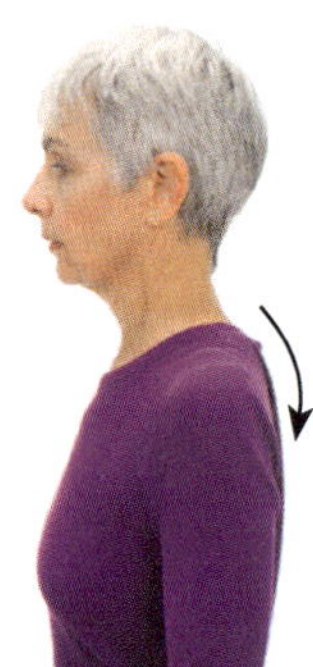

Figure 7

- Bring one shoulder forward *(figure 5)*, up *(figure 6)*, back, wide, and down *(figure 7)*. Repeat with the other shoulder. Let your arms be heavy.
- Back up your neck and your chin will move toward your throat. Look straight ahead.
- Stand tall. Follow the line between your heels and the crown of your head. Relax everywhere.

SIT A LITTLE

"Sit a little" while standing is a reminder to let the pelvis relax downward in front. Imagine sitting on the edge of a high stool, then keeping your pelvis in that position as you stand. Or crouch a little, as if you were about to jump. Either way, you will feel as though you are slightly seated.

CHECK AND FEEL

☑ *Do you feel weight in your heels?*

If not, crouch a little, into the position you would take instinctively if you were about to jump. Then straighten your knees, but keep the pelvis in its slightly seated position.

If you still feel weight in the front of your feet, "sit" more. The thigh muscles stay loose.

☑ *Does your back feel strained?*

You are probably lifting your chest. Let your ribs drop downward until your back muscles feel soft to the touch. Breathe into the lumbar spine to help relax that area.

IN BALANCE, STANDING WITH EASE

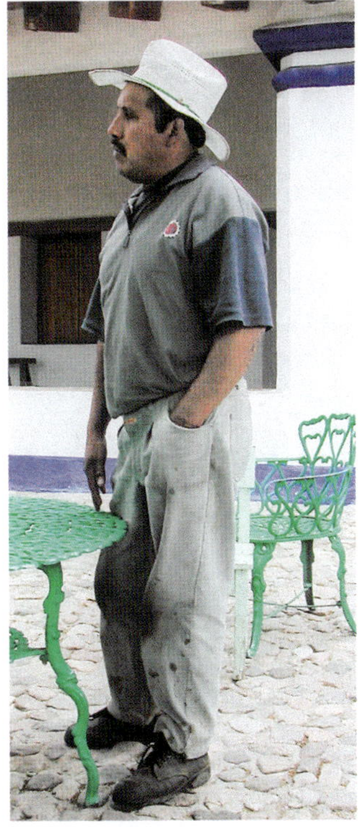

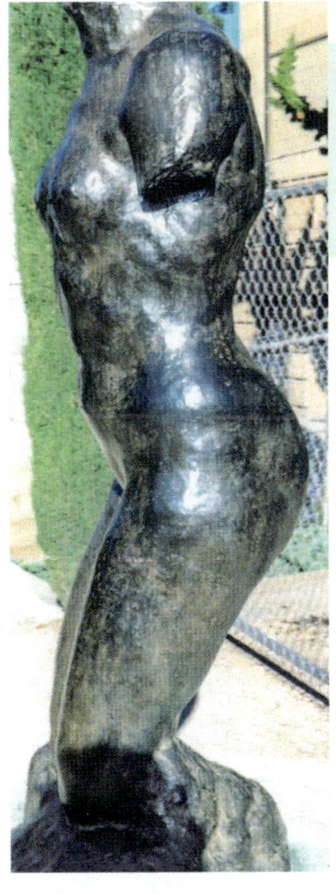

The man stands slightly seated, knees soft, and perfectly aligned. All in a natural, relaxed way. The statue in the center is slightly seated. At right, the feet are in a **V.**

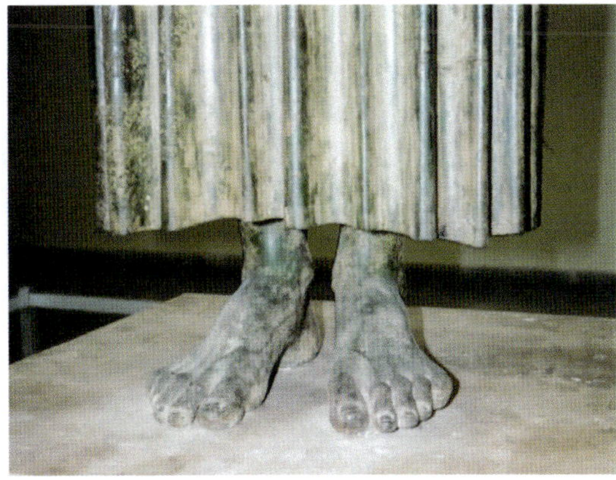

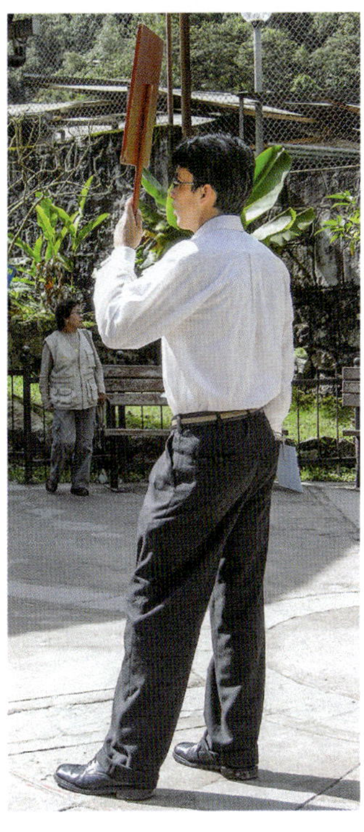

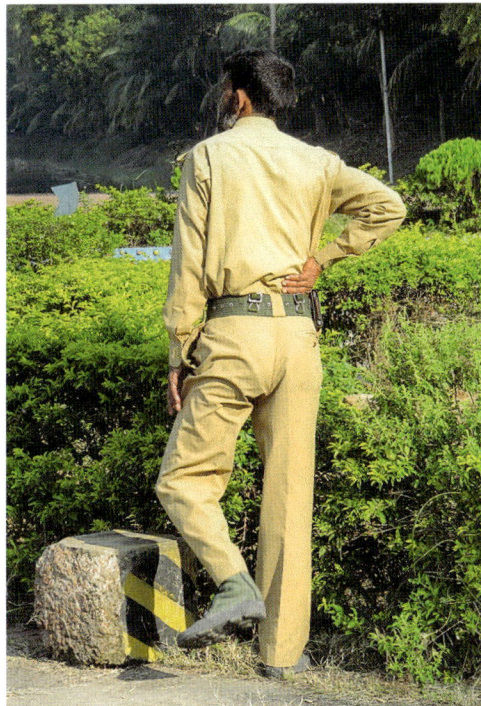

(Left) The Peruvian man, carrying a sign for arriving tourists, looks planted here. He stayed comfortably in this position for a long time without moving. Notice that his buttocks are behind him, as if he is very slightly seated.

(Right) When lifting one leg there is no need to lean to one side; the hips stay even.

Strengthening Your Feet

In many countries it is normal to stand or walk barefoot, or wear light flip-flops or other minimal shoes, even on rough terrain.

In Western cultures our feet have become accustomed to cushioning or constraint—layers of padding in tennis shoes, for example, so we don't feel the ground, or fashionable shoes with narrow toes. As the modern spine became more curved, weight distribution shifted so that the front of the foot now carries more of a burden than it was designed to do. Foot pain is common, even debilitating.

Healthy feet have a huge impact on the alignment of the entire skeleton. When you stand with your bones and joints aligned, weight reaches your feet in a straight line down your legs, and you will feel most of your weight in your heels. If your body is out of alignment, your weight is mostly in the front of your feet, your arches are flat, and *every joint in your body is slightly off-center.*

Shifting your body weight from the front of your feet into your heel bones is the single most important thing you can do for foot health. It will revitalize your feet and make them active participants in standing and walking. This is the secret to healthy feet.

In Balance. When you stand with your bones and joints aligned, weight reaches your feet in a straight line down your leg. You will feel about 80 percent of your weight in the back of your heel, 15 percent at the base of the big toe (at the metatarsal joint), and 5 percent in the tip of the big toe.

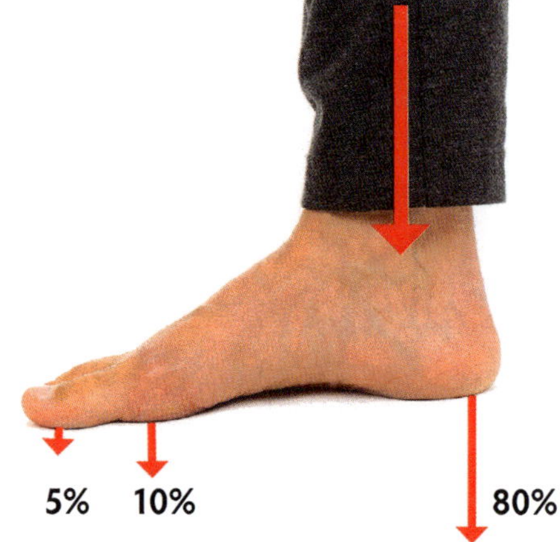

PUTTING WEIGHT IN YOUR HEELS

- Stand as you normally do and feel where your feet have weight. The weight is probably in the front, under the toes and ball of the foot.
- Now move the tops of your legs back until you feel weight in the center of your heels. You will have to sit a little to keep your balance and not let your toes come off the floor.
- Once you feel weight in your heels you may also notice that the arches are now lifted—your legs are now aligned with your pelvis and spine.

The task ahead is to get comfortable in this position and change the habit of leaning back when you walk or stand.

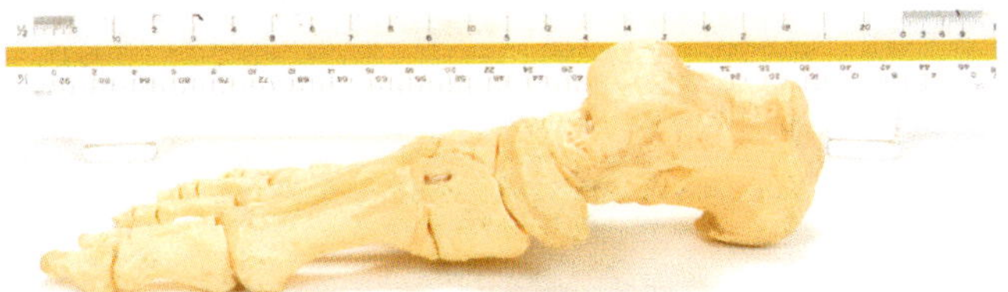

Flat arches

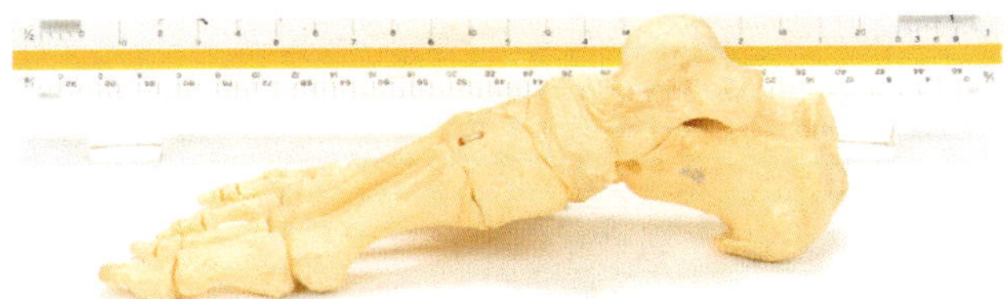

Lifted arches

Notice the difference in foot length (at least one shoe size) when arches are flat versus lifted.

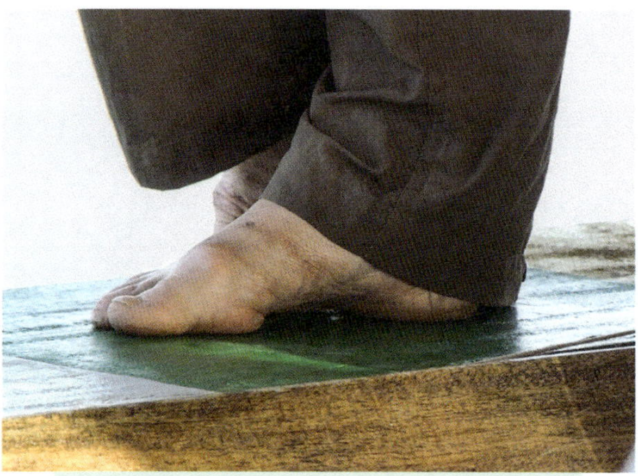

In Balance. In strong, healthy feet the foot slopes down toward the toes because the inner arches are lifted.

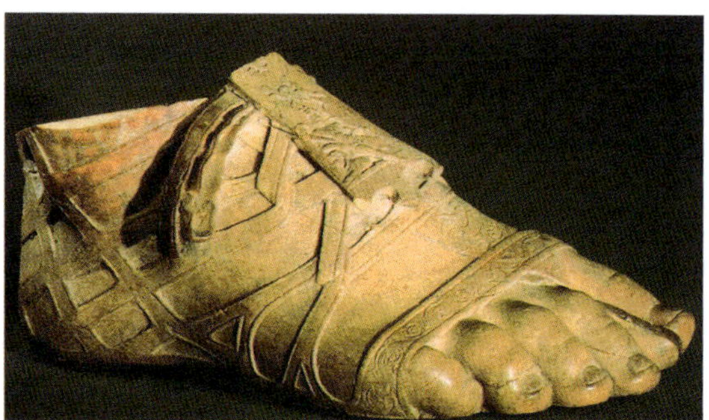

In Balance. The foot slopes down and the toe tips rest on the floor. Notice the slight lift of the outer arch along the outside edge of the foot.

ARCHES OF THE FOOT

The foot has three arches: Two are longitudinal and one is transverse.

The medial, inner arch is the highest and characteristic of flat feet when collapsed. In healthy feet it is well defined.

The lateral, outer arch is often collapsed as well when too much weight is carried on the outer edge of the foot. A flattening of the top of the outer foot is a visible sign of collapse.

The transverse arch runs across the mid-foot. When the foot does not slope down, but flattens just above the toes, this arch is collapsed.

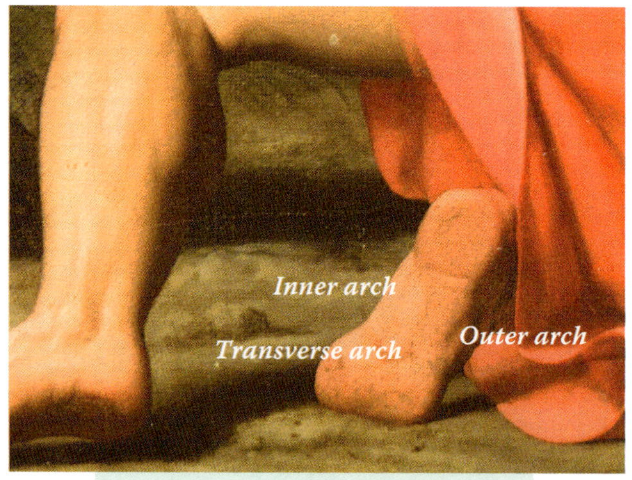

In Balance. Here the arches are well defined. On the left foot, note the slope from the upper part of the foot to the toes. On the right foot, note the muscular divide between inner and outer arches. (Detail from *Moses Defending the Daughters of Jethro* by Nicolas Colombel, c. 1686)

CARING FOR YOUR FEET

Massage

To lubricate the many foot joints it is helpful to massage them. Acupressure-like massage with a small cork ball under the metatarsal joints and the cuboid bones of the midfoot is helpful to restore and maintain vibrant feet.

If your feet are very sensitive, use a tennis ball at first. Gradually move to a harder, smaller ball.

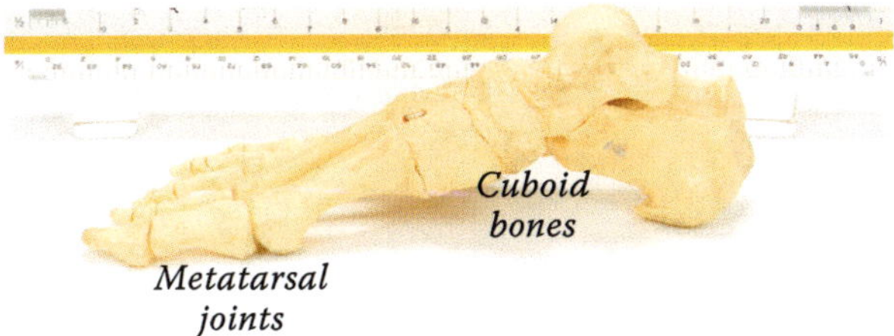

Foot-shortening exercise

This exercise will strengthen your arches and help your feet become active participants in standing and walking. While walking, the foot contracts in this position *at the moment of forward propulsion*, as you will see in the section on Walking.

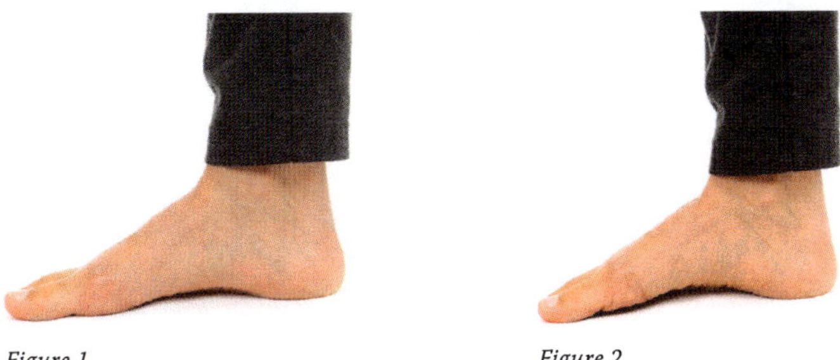

Figure 1 *Figure 2*

- Stand and focus on one foot. Keep the toe tips resting on the floor and weight in the center of the heel *(figure 1)*.
- Anchor the heel and gently press the tips of the toes down *(figure 2)*. This contracts the muscles under your foot, lifting the arches and shortening the foot. Your toes are relaxed; they do not tense or grip.
- Make sure that your foot is balanced so that weight is carried in the center of the heel. You will feel both the inner and outer arches contract.

- Hold and then release. Make this a gentle effort.
- Do this exercise while standing in line, or even while sitting in a chair.

CHECK AND FEEL

☑ *Is it difficult to keep weight in your heels?*

The weight will stay in your heels only as long as you stand in Balance, slightly seated. The moment you move away from this alignment, your weight will move to the front of your feet. It is helpful to feel the sensation of solid legs when weight moves down your leg bones into your heels.

BENDING, LIFTING, AND CARRYING IN BALANCE

We stand looking at half a dozen women working, bent double, knees straight: impossible to work like this, you think, but they do, for hours. Their feet bare, because of the mud.

~ Doris Lessing[17]

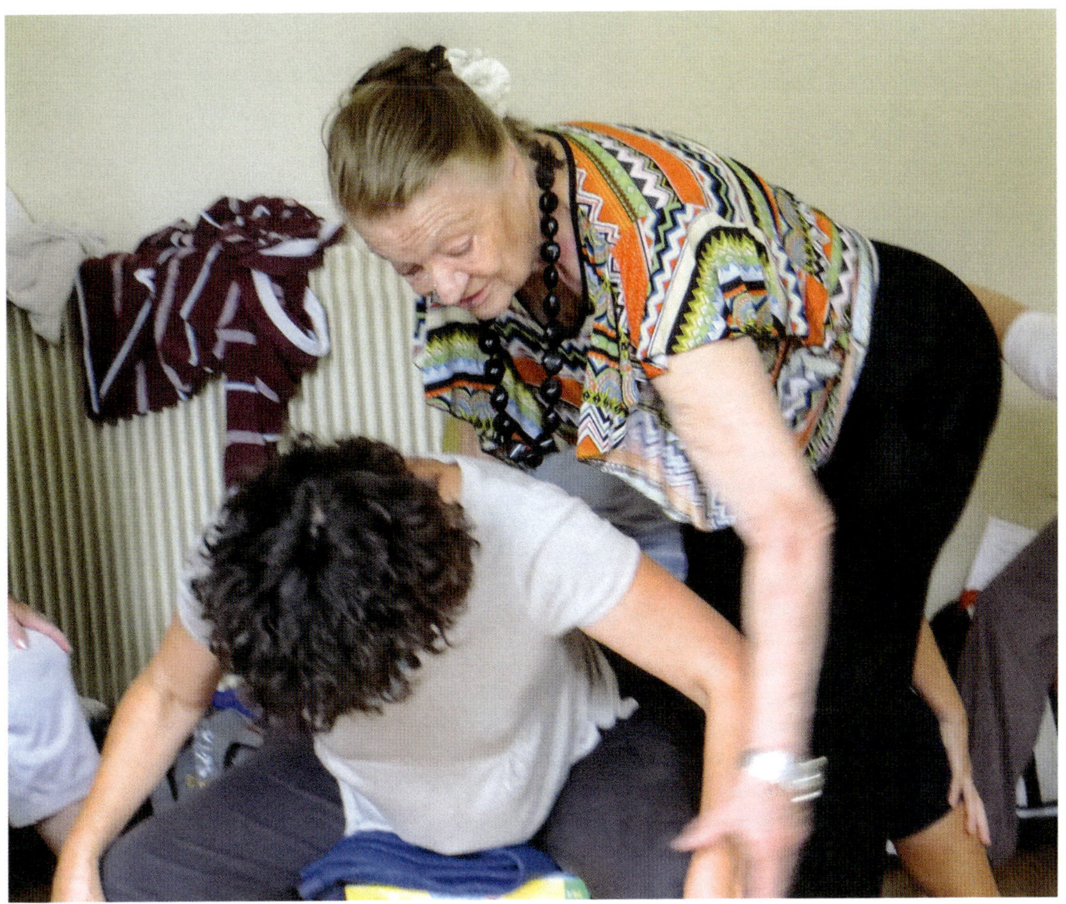

Noëlle Perez-Christiaens teaching at age 86. She bends with ease and a straight back.

Bending

HINGE AT THE HIPS

"Hinge at the hips" is a reminder to bend from the hip joints, not from the waist, and with a straight back. Whenever you bend, pivot from your hips and keep your back from rounding. This is the secret to bending safely.

Bending in Balance means bending at the hip joints, with a flat back. The hip joint is the hinge that enables the lifting and lowering of the trunk over the legs. Not only is this way of bending safe, it also keeps the joints mobile and the muscles supple.

It is important to understand the difference between bending at the hip joints and bending at the waist. If you bend at the waist—right above your hip bones, at the height of a belt—you are forced to round your back because the spine is not designed to bend at the waist. If you bend at the hip joints, the spine has no need to round. It bends safely.

Bending at the hip joints and keeping your back straight is the *single most important thing you can do* to prevent back pain and injury.

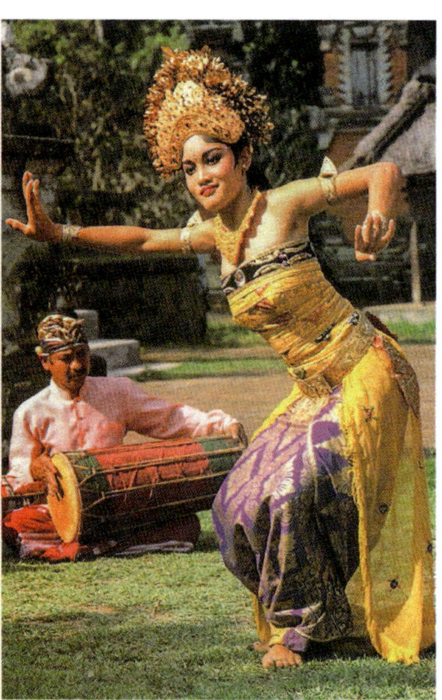

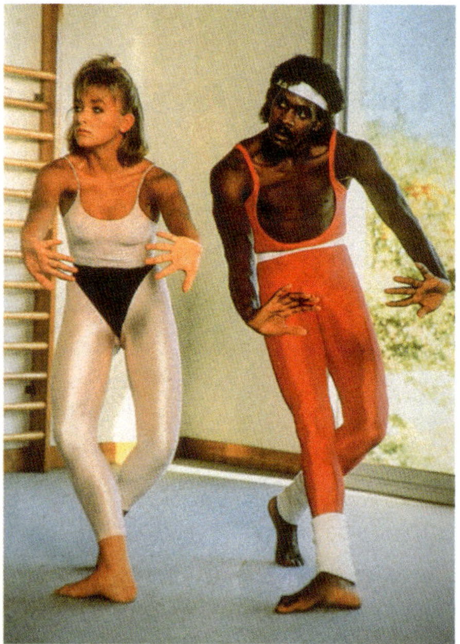

(Left) **In Balance.** This traditional Indonesian dancer bends at the hips. Notice the long torso and low belt, at the natural arch. (Right) **Out of Balance.** Modern dancers bending at the waist.

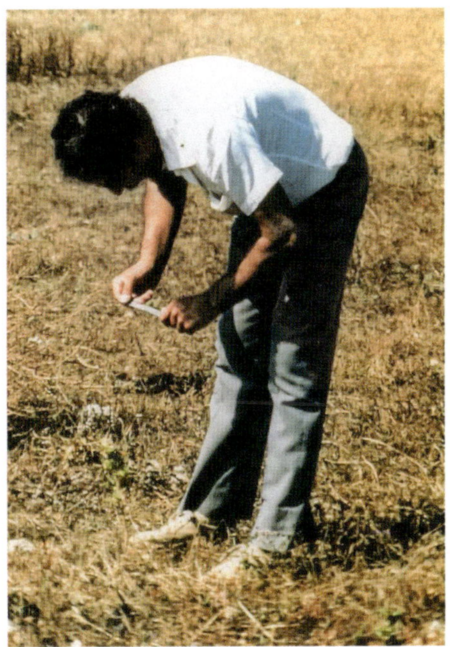

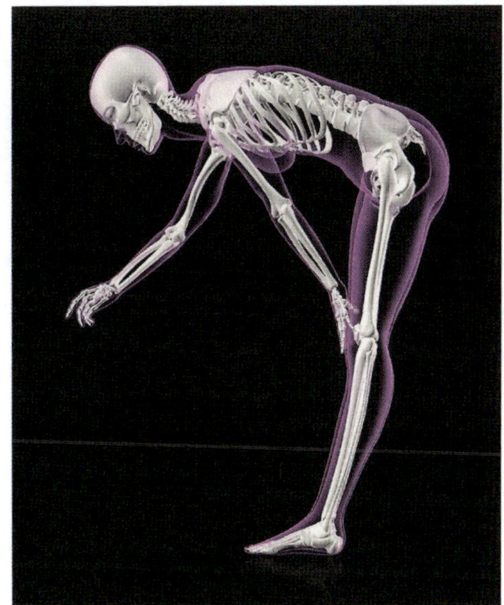

Out of Balance. Bending from the waist. The hips, knees, and ankles are locked and pushed back—visible in the man's knees and the skeleton. Bending this way forces the back to round and the neck to arch.

In Balance. Miguel bends from the hips with legs wide, knees bent and aligned over the feet, and a flat back. The buttocks lift, visible in the upward stretch of his pants.

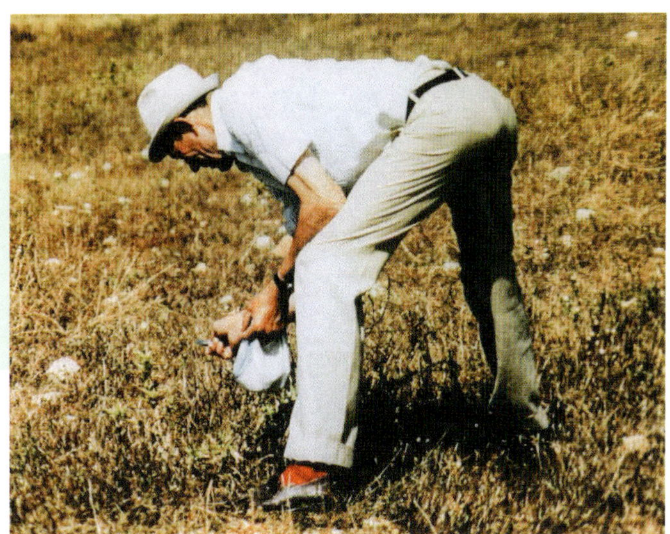

Out of Balance. Bending with a rounded spine places this man at high risk for damage to disks and joints.

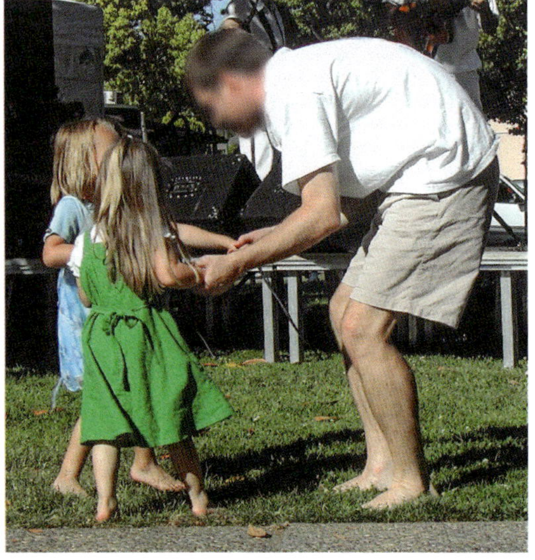

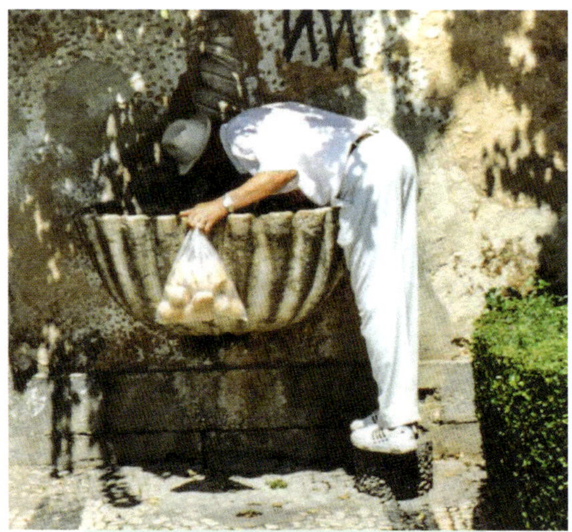

In Balance. Hinging at the hips with a flat spine.

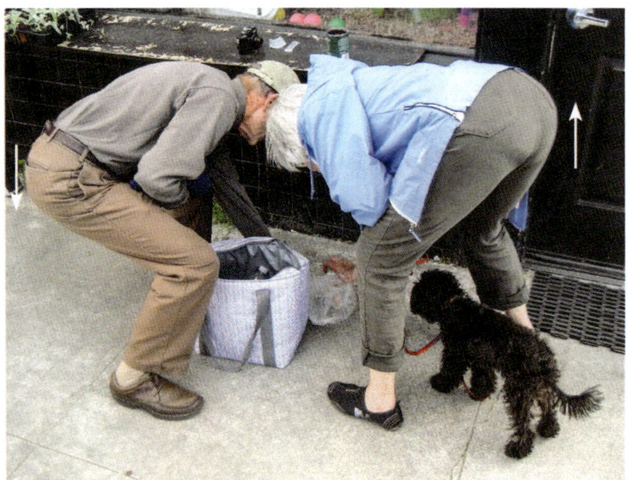

Out of Balance. The person at left squats, which requires his back to round.

In Balance. In contrast, the person at right lifts her buttocks, which puts the pelvis in a forward-rotated position and allows the back to stay flat.

In Balance. Bend by hinging at the hips and keeping the back flat, whether you bend from a seated or a standing position.

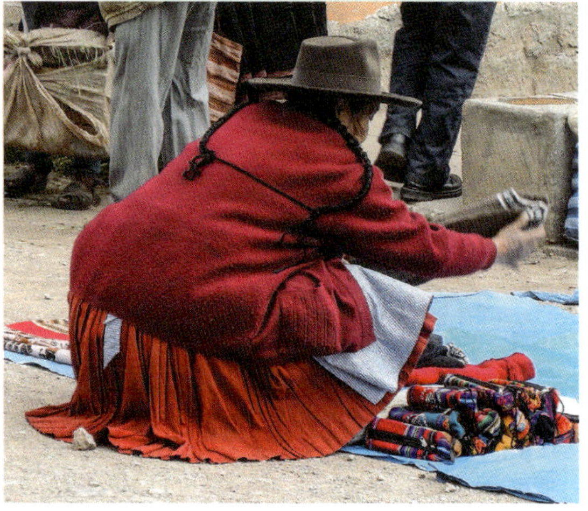

Follow the practice guidelines below and become aware of the sensations in your hips, back, legs, and feet. Each time you bend is an opportunity to stretch your hamstrings, mobilize your hip joints, and relax your low back. No need to go to the gym!

If your hamstrings are tight, you will need to bend your knees more. With repetition your hamstrings will elongate, little by little, and you will feel very comfortable bending in this way.

HOW TO PRACTICE

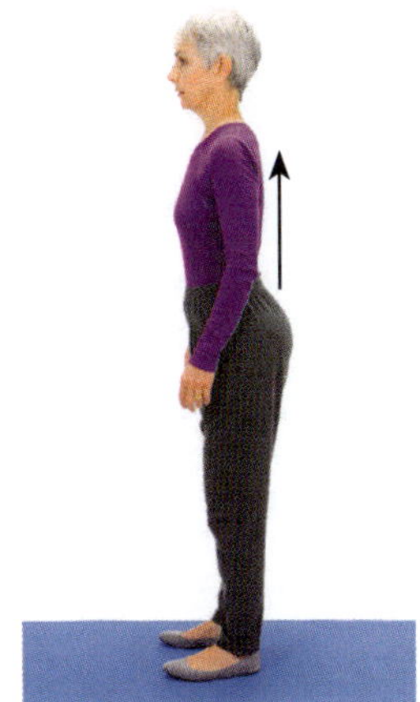

Figure 1

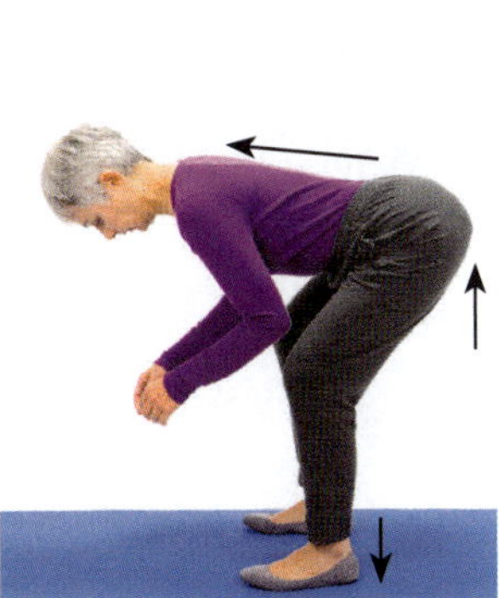

Figure 2

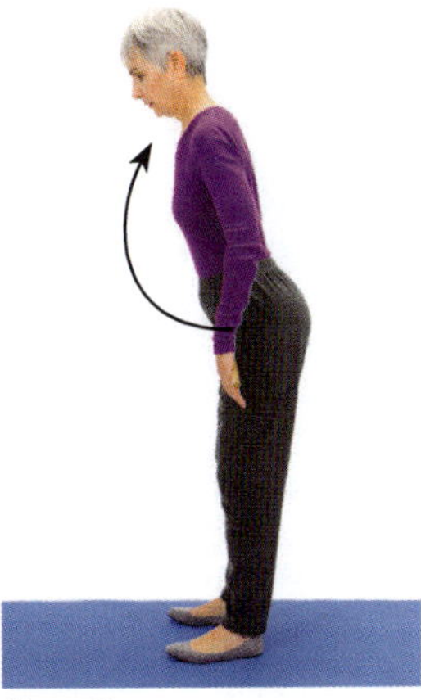

Figure 3

- Place your legs a little wider apart than for standing, knees soft and feet in a slight **V.** Relax your belly and back. Lift and extend the spine, feeling weight in your heels *(figure 1).*
- Tip your torso forward like a jackknife, hinging at your hip sockets and taking your sitting bones skyward. Let your spine move as a unit, like a yardstick, neither arching nor rounding your back. Let your knees bend wide over your feet, on the median line. *Keep weight in your heels (figure 2).*
- Feel a stretch in your hamstrings and buttock muscles.
- To come up, unhinge at your hip sockets and at the same time straighten your legs—always with a sensation of lightness *(figure 3).*

CHECK AND FEEL

DEEP BENDING

For a deep bend, place your feet wide with knees centered over the feet. Your knees may be in front of your ankles, but should not be out in front of your feet. Your buttocks should be well behind you.

The deeper the bend, the higher the buttocks must lift to prevent the back from rounding. This requires a smooth interplay between muscles and joints. The knees, hips, and ankles must balance each other, flexing just the right amount, and the leg muscles must make it possible.

When any one of the parts involved is out of alignment or stiff, we compensate by bending in ways that cause damage and pain. Learning to bend properly is critical.

☑ *Does your weight stay in your heels?*

Most people have tight hamstrings that pull the pelvis down in back. (Your hamstrings are on the back of your thighs.) When your hamstrings tighten you will no longer feel weight in your heels. The moment you feel your hamstrings tighten, bend your knees just enough to keep weight in your heels. But don't let your knees come forward, in front of your ankles. Remember, the main hinge is at the hips—rotate there!

Visualize length in the back of your legs as your tailbone rises.

☑ *Does your low back feel tight?*

Your low back is probably arched and if you place your hand there you can feel a hollow. Start over and become aware of the habit of lifting your chest and arching your low back as you bend.

Stand and drop your chest, relaxing your low back and keeping it relaxed as you rotate at your hip joints. Weight stays in your heels.

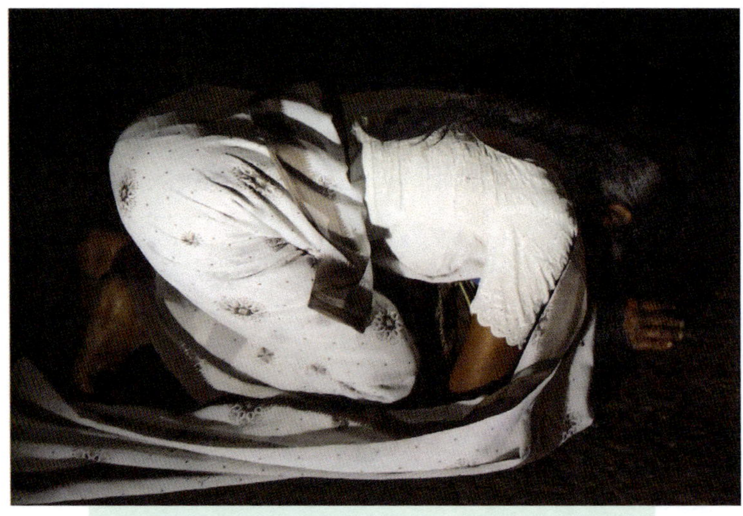

In Balance. In bending, the main hinge is at the hips. In a deep bend the tailbone points back at an acute angle. Miguel compares this point to a bird's beak. The closer you get to this shape, the more you are rotating the pelvis at the hip joints.

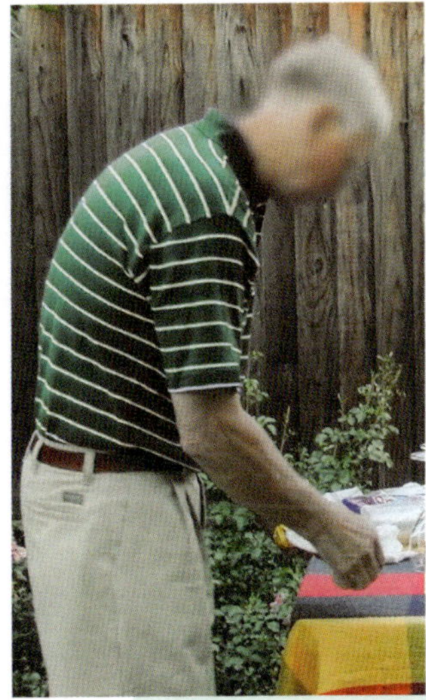

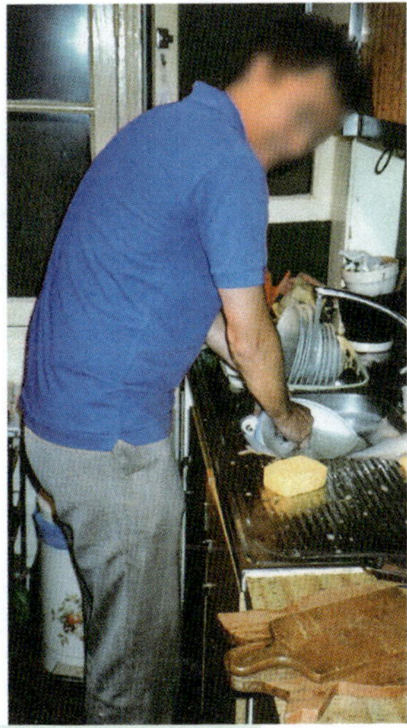

Out of Balance. Common ways of bending with a rounded upper back.

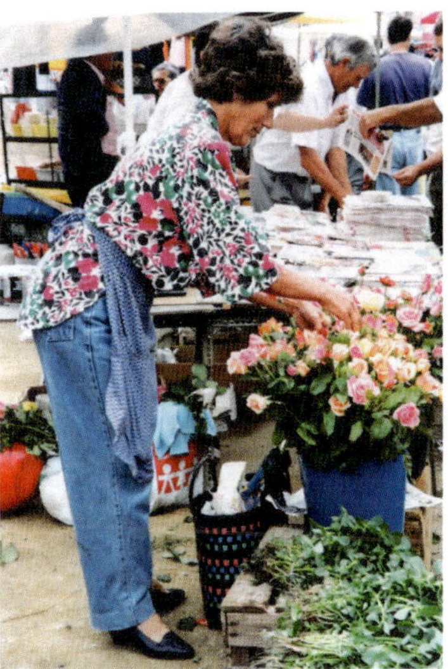

In Balance. Bending from the hips with a flat back.

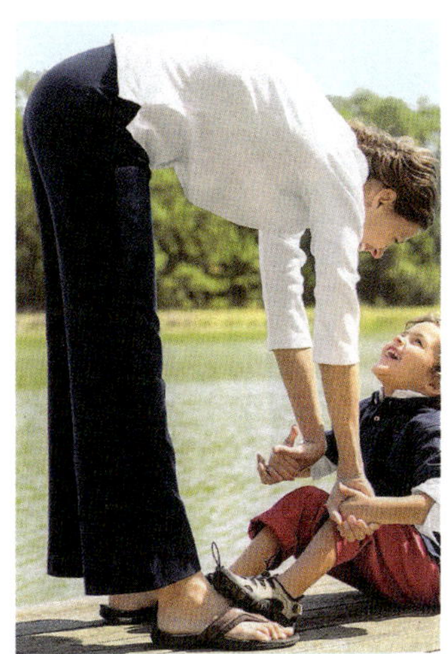

Out of Balance. This woman bends deeply but locks her knees and hips. She bends as little as possible at her hips, so her spine has to round.

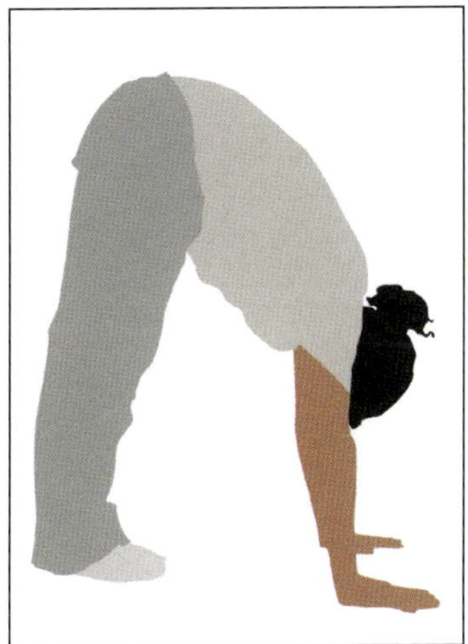

Out of Balance. Knees are locked and the hips are not bent enough. The back rounds to compensate.

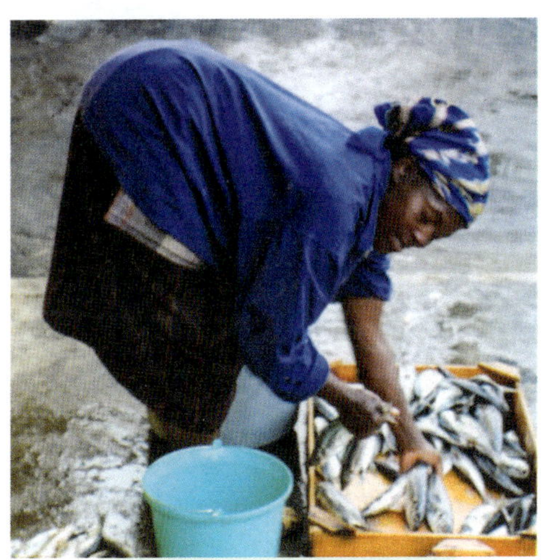

In Balance. In this deep bend, the knees are not locked but slightly bent, and the hips bend deeply so that the back is free to extend in a straight line.

There are so many opportunities to bend.
To reach...

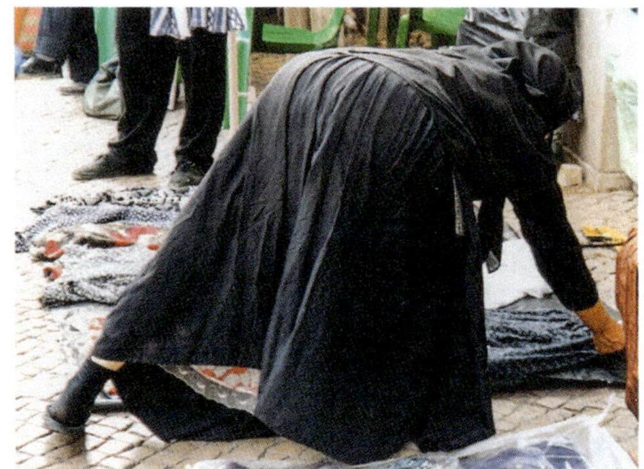

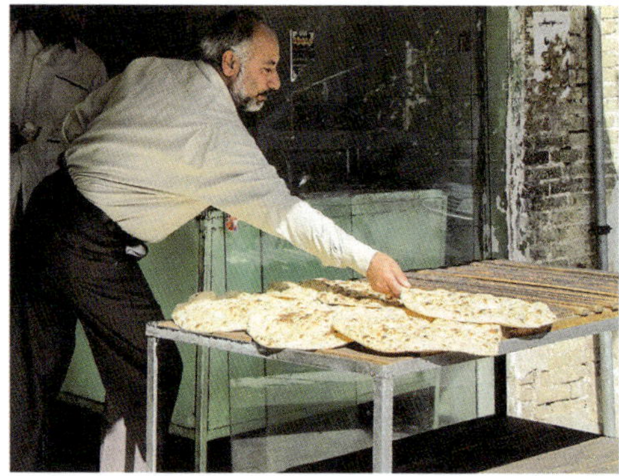

to talk to someone seated...

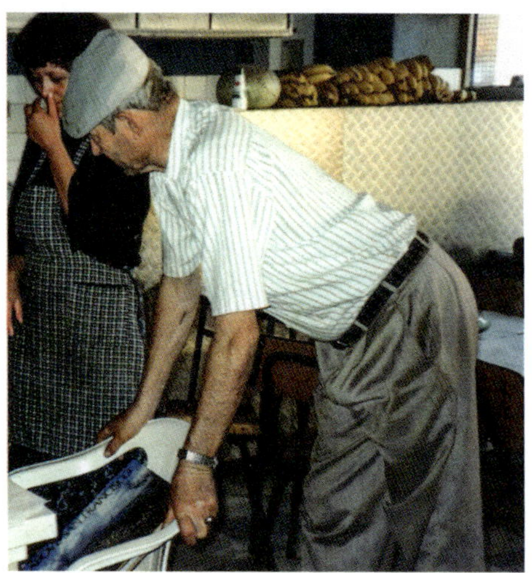

to push off...

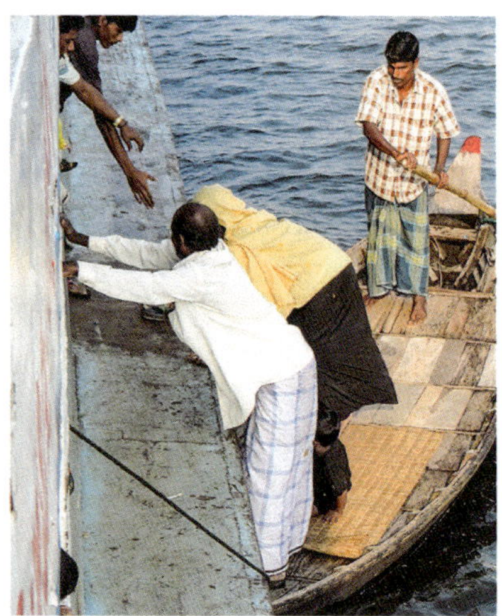

to garden.

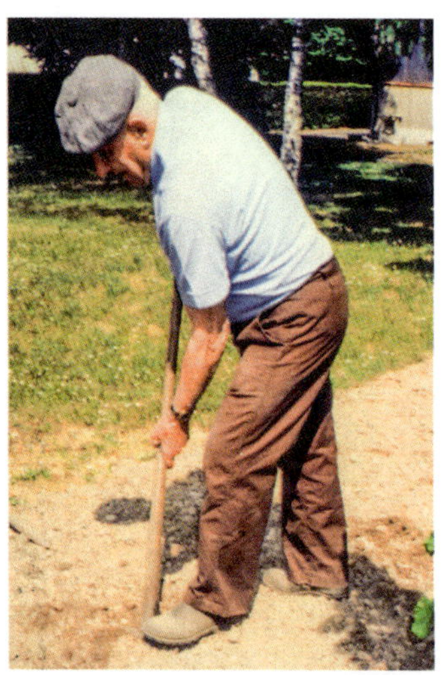

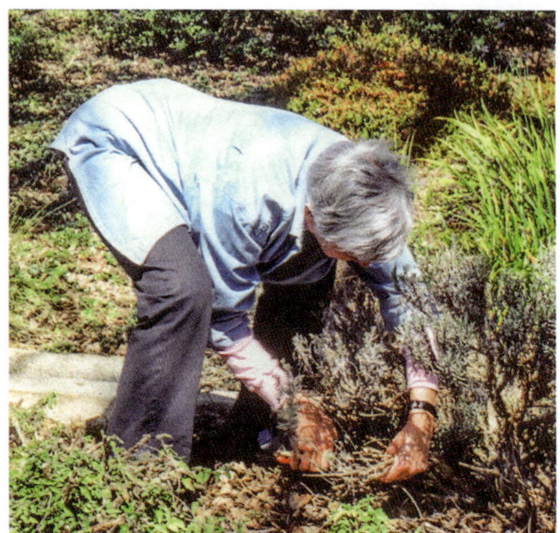

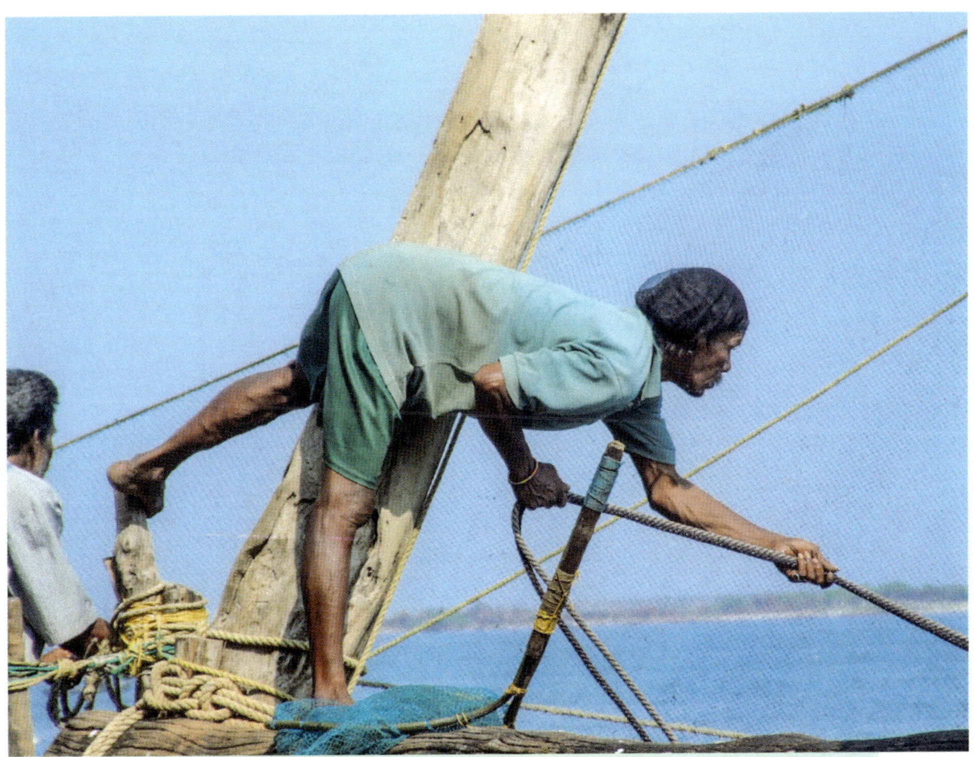

In Balance. Bending takes many forms, but the same principles apply. This man's habit of bending at the hips with a flat back has allowed him to maintain natural alignment and strength. He stands firmly on one leg, using his other leg to steady himself as he works. His front leg is strong as a post.

Lifting

To lift you will need to bend. The same principles apply as for bending: Hinge at the hips and keep the back flat. The practice guidelines show you how to lift safely.

In Balance. The buttocks are behind the legs, weight is in the heels, and knees are wide.

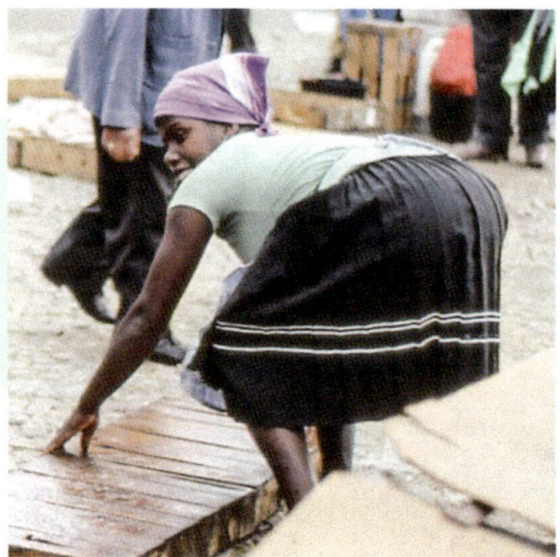

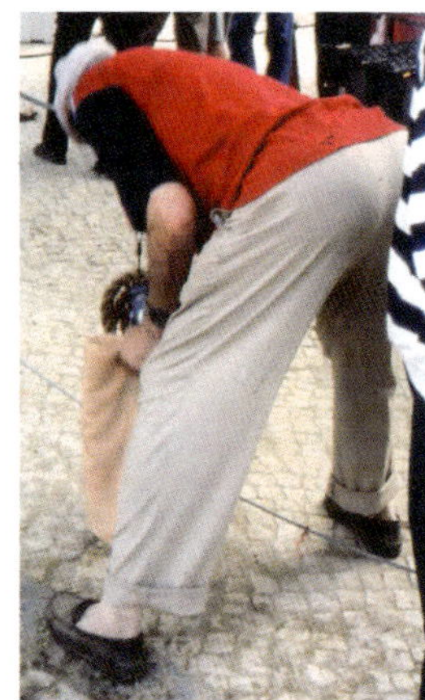

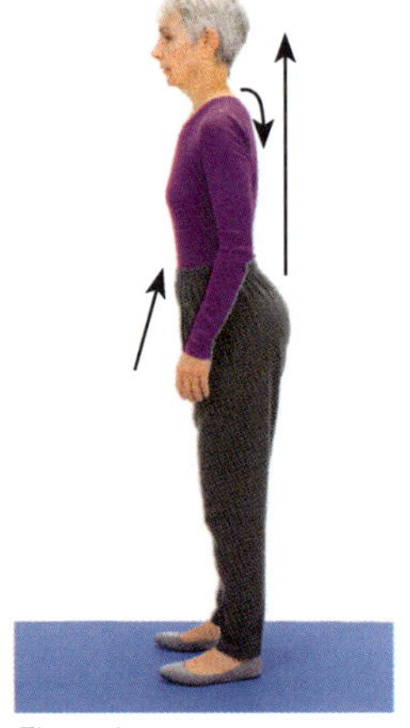

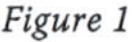

Figure 1

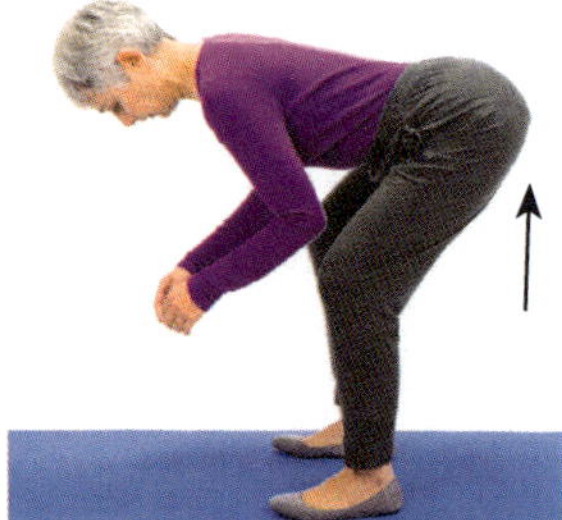

Figure 2

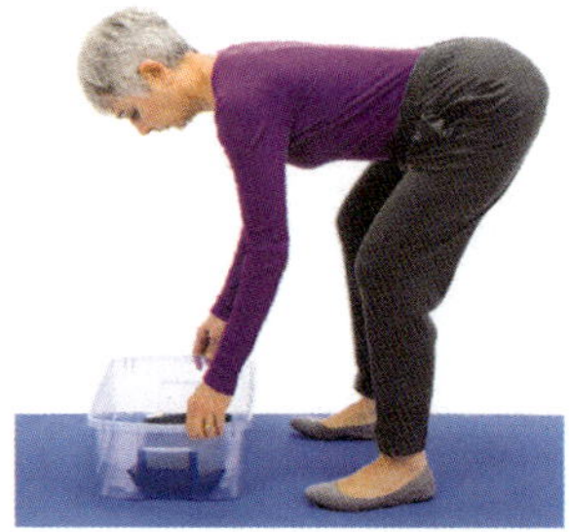

Figure 3

HOW TO PRACTICE

- Take a wide stance.
- Lengthen your spine and engage the corselet. Feel your stomach draw up and in as your spine extends. Draw one shoulder at a time back and down *(figure 1).*
- Tip your torso forward, hinging at your hip sockets and taking your sitting bones skyward. Let your spine move as a unit, like a yardstick, neither arching nor rounding your back. To get down low, bend your knees wide over your feet, *knees barely in front of your toes (figure 2).*

- Take hold of the object, which should be placed close to you *(figure 3)*.

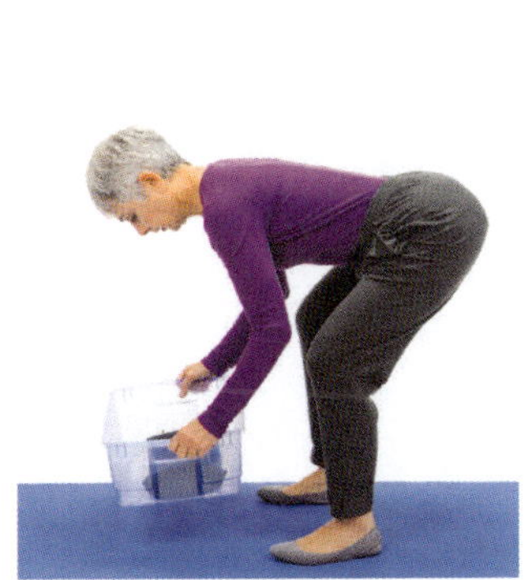

Figure 4

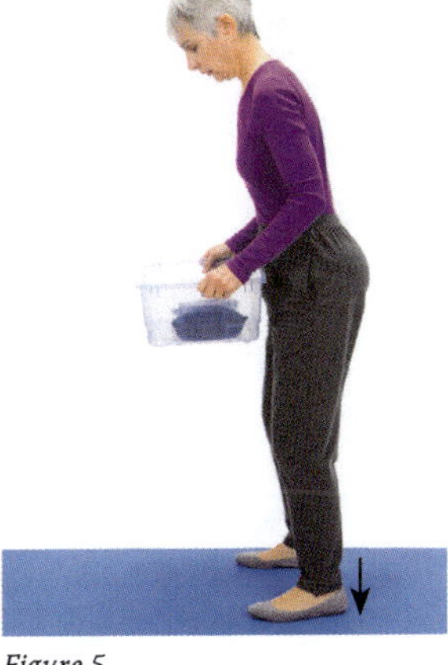

Figure 5

CAUTION!

The lifting action is in your legs and corselet muscles. If your back hurts while lifting or bending, stop! Contact a Balance instructor for guidance. Do not lift anything heavy until you understand how to lift safely and without pain.

- To lift, come up by pressing down on your heels as you straighten your knees and hips. The corselet stays active the whole time to prevent your back from arching *(figure 4)*.
- Resist the urge to pull the weight of the object up with your arms. Let your legs straighten, while holding the object close to your body. The legs do the lifting *(figure 5)*.

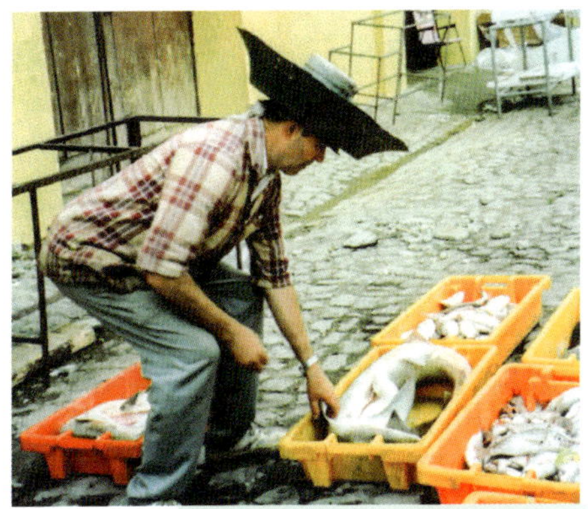

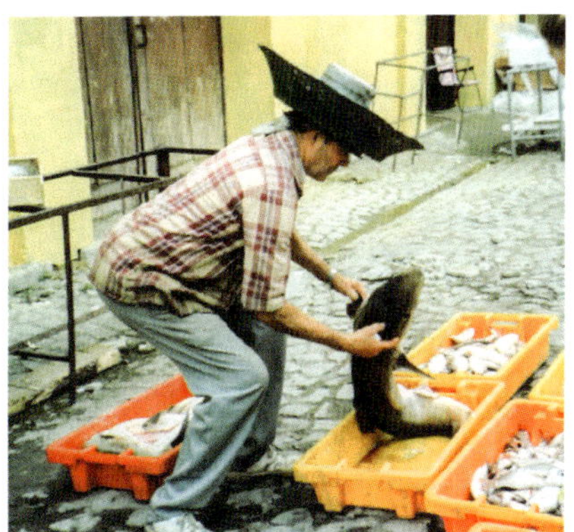

In Balance. Miguel bends to lift a heavy fish. First he brings the fish close, then lifts by straightening his legs. The creases in his pants (right) indicate an upward lift in his buttocks and the back of the legs as he straightens. His back remains flat.

Carrying

There are many ways to carry, but the same rule applies to all: Let the front of the pelvis stay down (fig) and engage your corselet muscles to lift and keep your weight centered.

In Balance. The corselet action of the abdominal muscles is clearly visible.

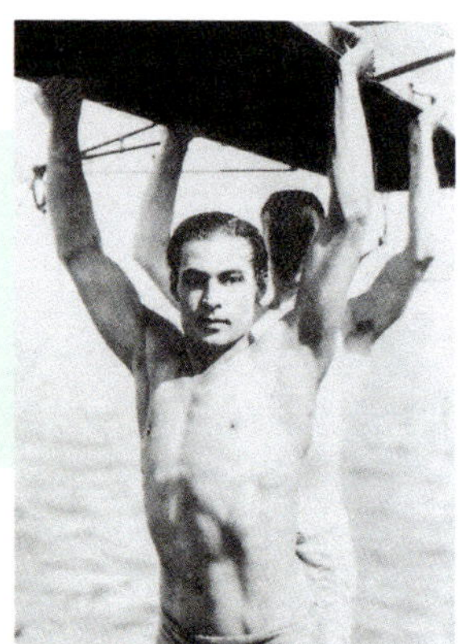

HOW TO CARRY A SHOULDER BAG

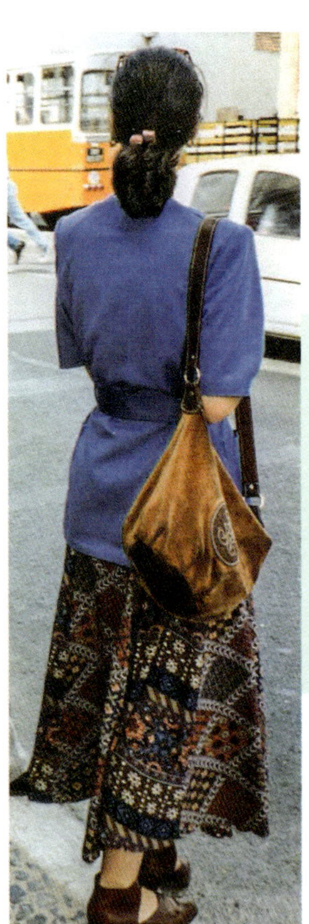

When carrying a shoulder bag it is common to lift your shoulder on the bag side of your body. Instead, lift along the median line to center your weight. If this is difficult, carry the strap across your chest to distribute weight evenly over your trunk.

Which back can be divided into two symmetrical halves? The habit of lifting one shoulder to carry a bag causes serious misalignment, but the habit can be easy to change.

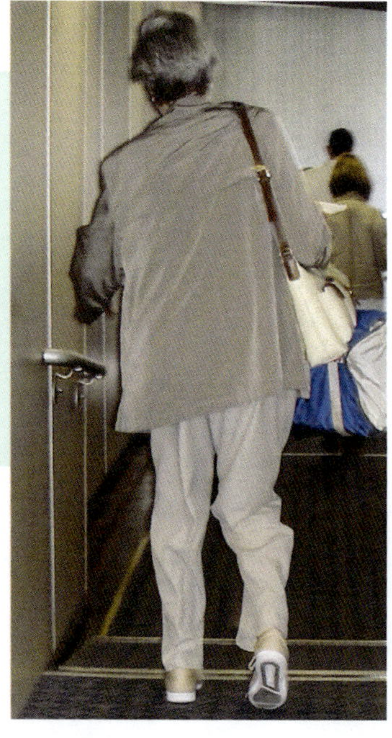

HOW TO CARRY WITHOUT LIFTING YOUR SHOULDERS

When you carry an object, keep your shoulders down. Notice the shoulders of the Peruvian woman at right, who is carrying bowls of hot soup. Her shoulders stay down, with the elbows directly underneath.

When you carry in this way, it is important to keep whatever you are carrying close to your body, so that:

- Your elbows can hug your sides
- Your shoulder blades slide down your back
- You lift up through your spine as you carry the weight

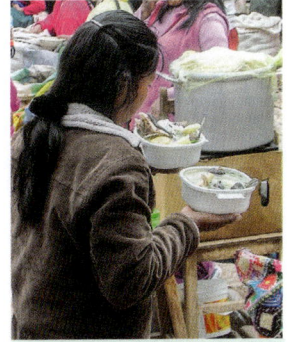

In Balance.
Shoulders are down and the elbows directly under them as this woman carries the bowls.

HOW TO CARRY A CHILD

The same principles apply to carrying a child: Lift up through the spine and stay tall. Do not lean or stoop. Visualize the distribution of weight along the vertical axis of gravity.

People in Balance carry children many different ways, but stay tall. They balance their weight, offsetting the weight of the child, without stooping or leaning to one side. There are some striking differences in how cultures other than our own carry children.

Most often, children are carried on the adult's back and with open legs. This benefits the child: The wide, open hips enable the child to develop the ability to squat and maintain a long spine. It also benefits the carrier: The child's weight rests on the strong bones of the pelvis, and the spine is in a slightly forward position that keeps it straight and not arched. The hands are free.

When carried in a sling, the child may ride on the hip, again of benefit as a hip-opener.

When carried in the arms, the child sits high with its head at the same level as or higher than the carrier's head (see photos on the next page, top left). This permits the carrier to stay tall and not let his or her shoulders come forward.

SUPPORTING OPEN HIPS AND A LONG SPINE

All healthy children up until the age of three or four are in Balance. But in Western culture they must conform to rounded car and stroller seats and are often carried with dangling, parallel legs. These positions fail to open the hips, rotate the pelvis forward, or lengthen the spine. As cartilage and bone develop they grow into a shape that is most comfortable in a rounded, closed (fetal) position. This gradual shaping, along with copying the posture of adults and older children around them, means that children lose the natural alignment they are born with.

CARRYING A CHILD IN BALANCE

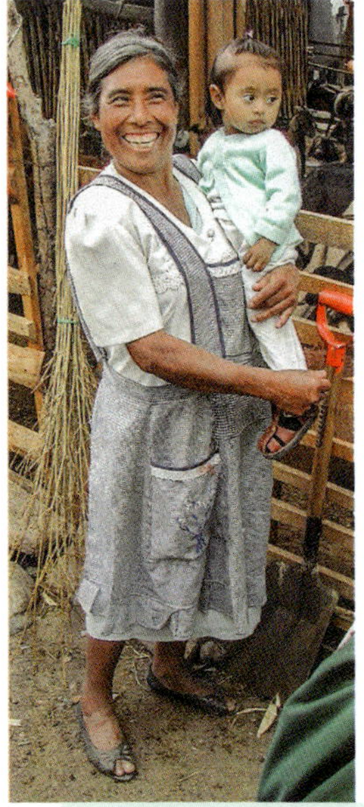

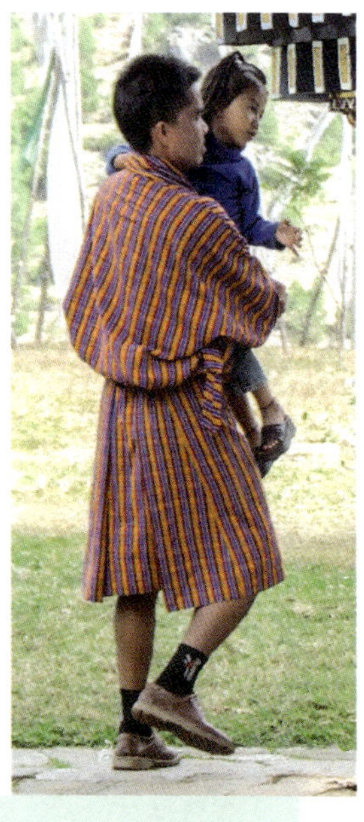

(Left) Notice the wide, open chest and vitality of this happy grandmother. Her shoulders are back and down and the child sits in the fold of her arm. (Right) An older child still carried high by her straight-backed dad.

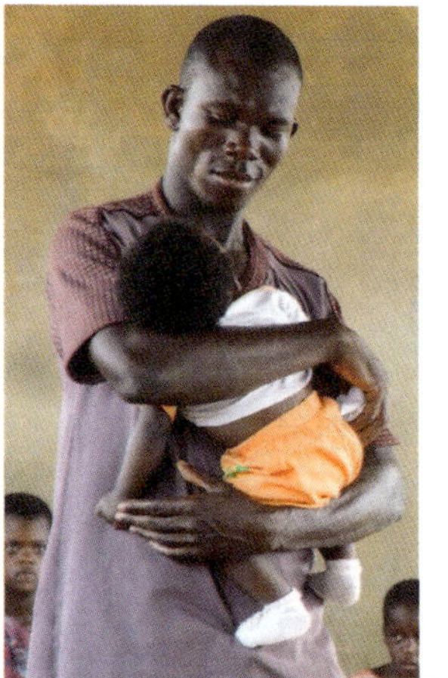

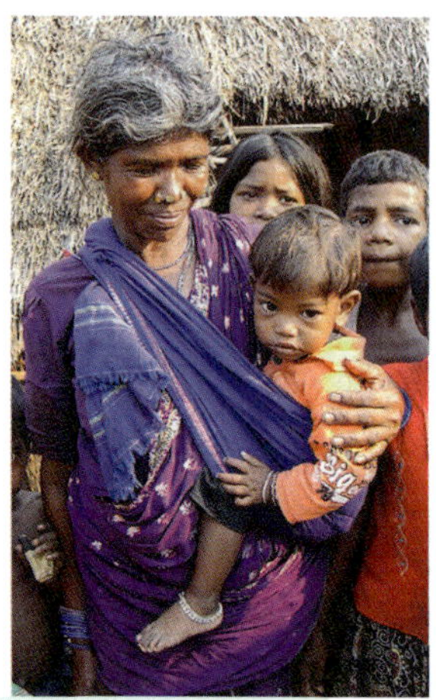

(Left) Notice how gently this sleeping child is held with both arms, each arm supporting a different part of the baby. The baby is held in a seated position. (Right) Well seated in a sling, legs apart.

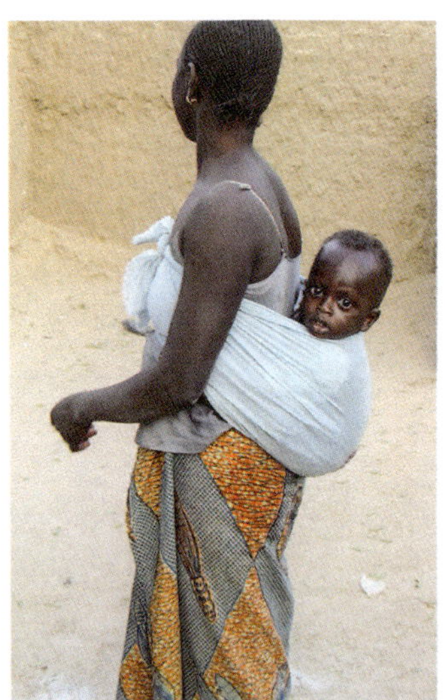

Carrying in Balance is graceful.

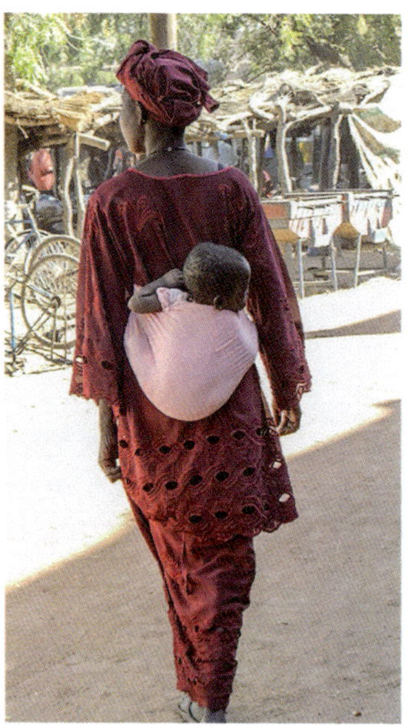

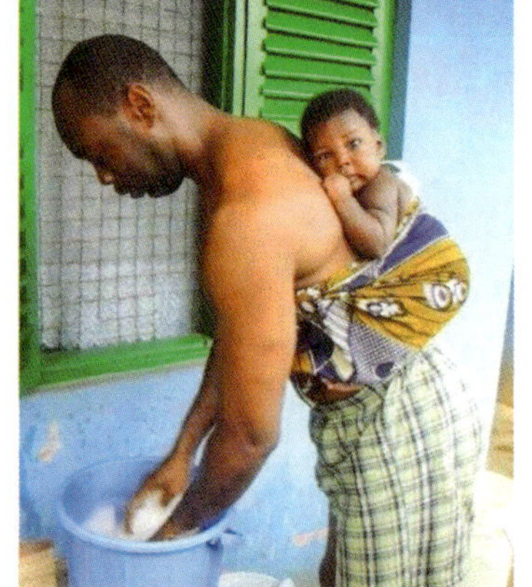

This child leans comfortably into the back of its dad, who has his hands free for the laundry.

WALKING IN BALANCE

Village women, walking tall as queens under the family wash balanced on their heads, waded across mud shallows to reach shallow pools.

~ Harriet Doerr[18]

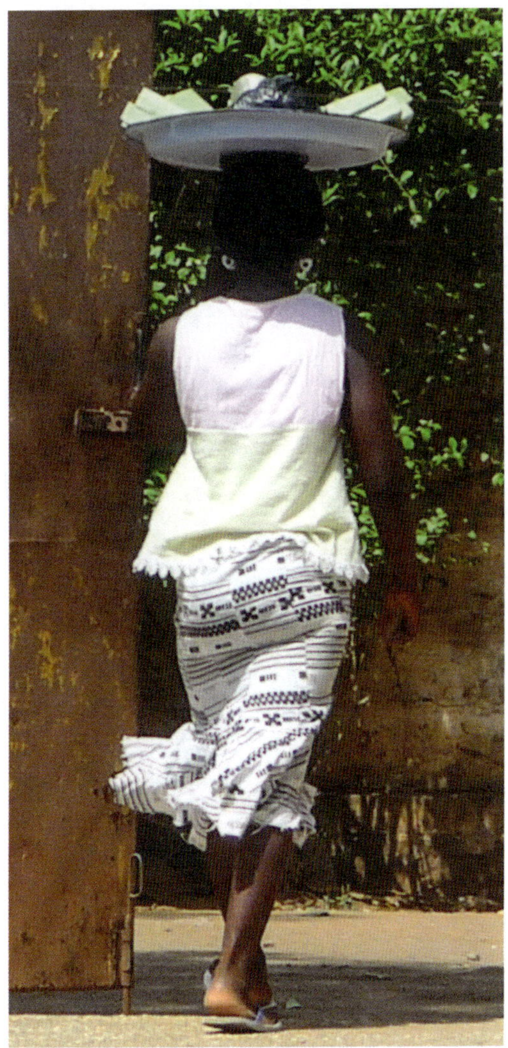

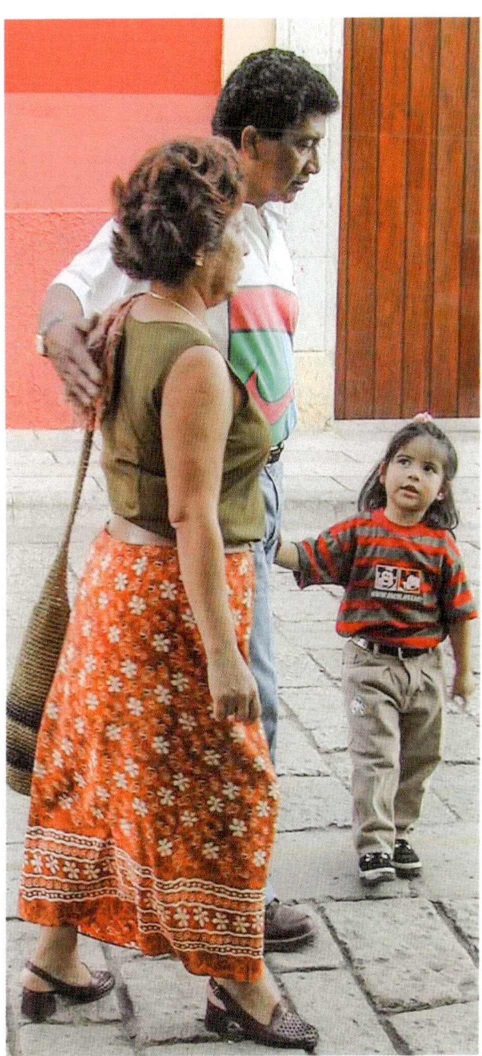

Walking naturally upright, in Balance. In midstep, both feet are on the ground.

Walking with Grace and Energy

In walking, everything you learned so far comes into play. The feet contract, the pelvis angles down in front, the abdominals engage, the spine and neck extend up, the shoulders relax, and the arms and legs swing freely.

The trunk and head stay quiet as the legs and feet move. The spine stays centered without swaying of the hips or zigzag twisting of the spine. All action is in the buttock muscles (the glutes, which include both the gluteus major and minor) and the feet.

In Balance. (Left) "Village women, walking tall as queens under the family wash...." (Right) Men as well look strong and graceful when they carry weight on their head.

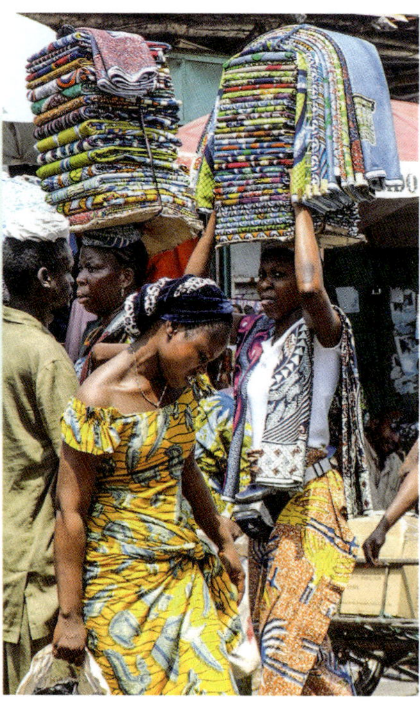

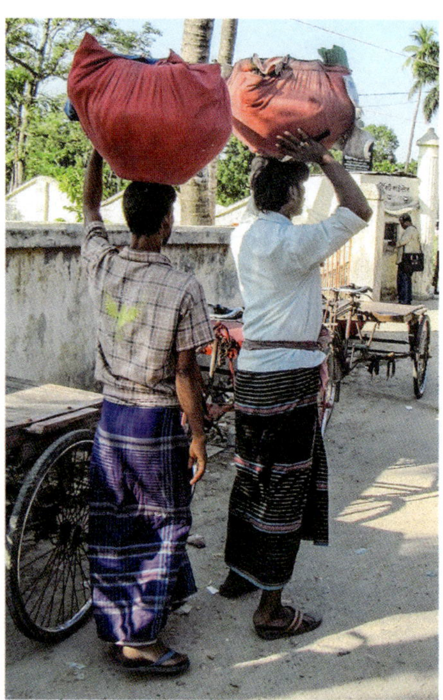

The walk of people in Balance is a light step—smooth, energetic, and soundless. When you walk behind a person like this you see clearly the strong muscle action in the buttocks. The person moves through space staying completely vertical, leaning neither forward nor backward.

To change the way you walk is no easy task. Walking is affected by culture, habit, and physical condition. Walking is complex. You will benefit from practicing with a Balance teacher.

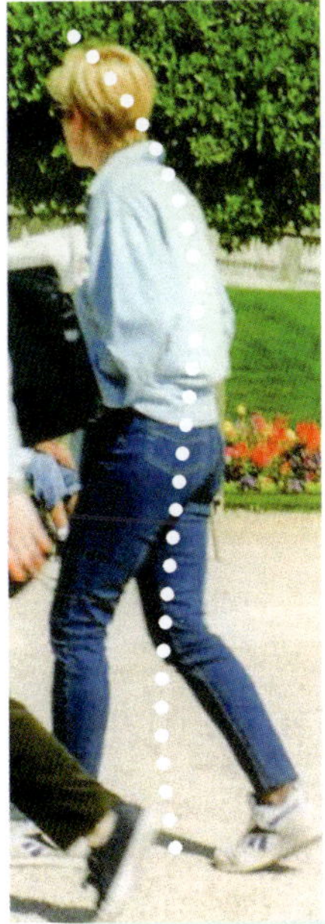

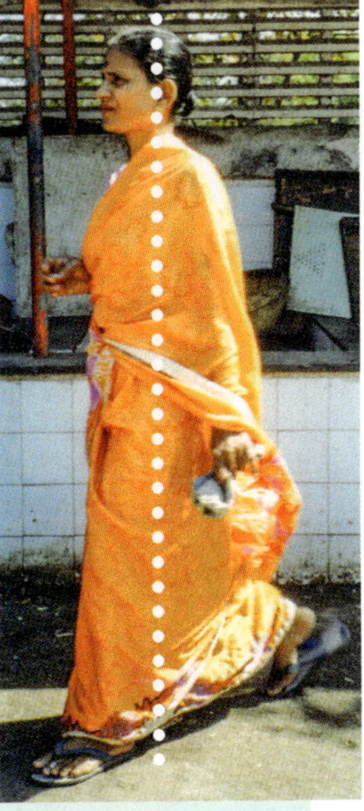

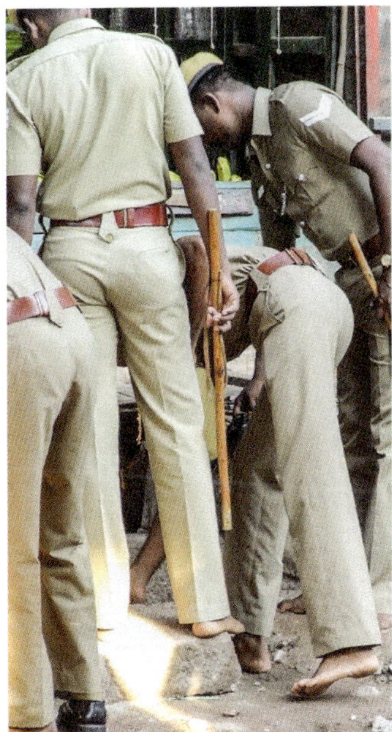

In Balance. Clearly visible, high buttock muscles at the base of the spine are due to strong muscle action during walking. This muscle development happens only when the pelvis is rotated down in front.

Notice the difference in energy and poise in these two women.

(Left) **Out of Balance.** The woman slumps as she walks. (Right) **In Balance.** The Indian woman stays perfectly upright as she walks. Until you look at her feet, she seems to be standing still. The back foot pushes off strongly.

To begin, it is helpful to break walking into components and practice each one separately before you try putting them all together:

1. Initiating a step
2. Pushing off with your back leg
3. Transferring your weight

HOW TO PRACTICE THE COMPONENTS OF WALKING

1. Initiating a step

- Stand in Balance, bent slightly at the hips as if sitting a little.
- Take a step back with your right leg, shifting all your weight onto this leg. You should be able to lift your left foot. Stay slightly seated.

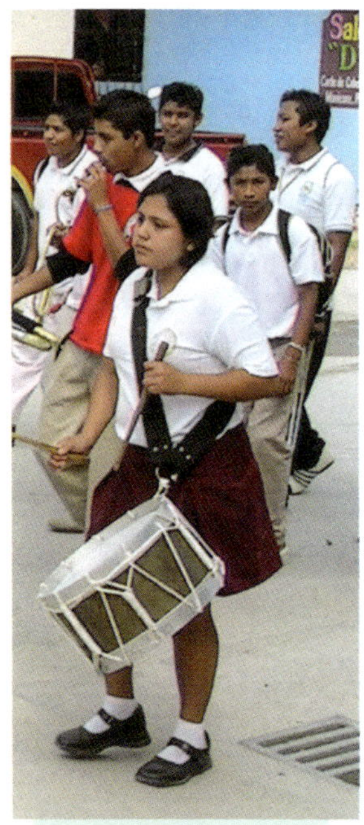

In Balance. The drummer girl has all her weight on the back leg (in this case the left leg), leaving the front leg free to swing. Notice the forward rotation of her pelvis.

- Your right leg feels strong and straight, weight in the heel, and ready for push-off.

2. P*ushing off with your back leg*

- Continue to focus on your right, weight-bearing leg. All the action is there.
- Lift your heel with a strong heel-to-toe contraction (as described in the Foot-shortening Exercise on page 73) and bend your knee. Your buttocks contract—they feel firm.
- Meanwhile, your left leg swings forward *on its own*, in tandem with the action of the right leg.
- Your right foot pushes off from the tips of the toes and weight transfers to the left leg.
- Keep your weight in the back leg *as long as possible!*

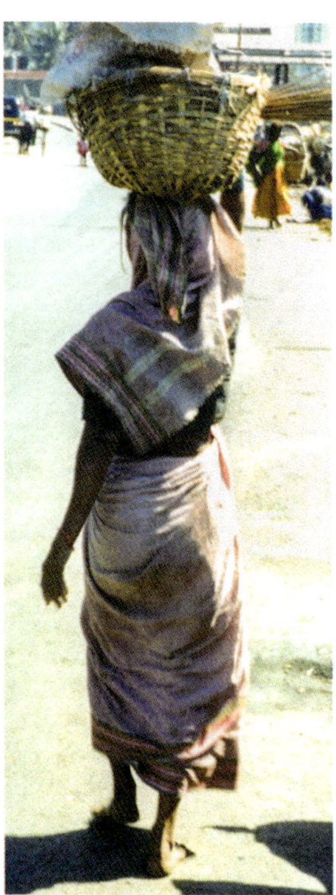

In Balance. All the weight is on the right (back) leg. The left foot is weightless.

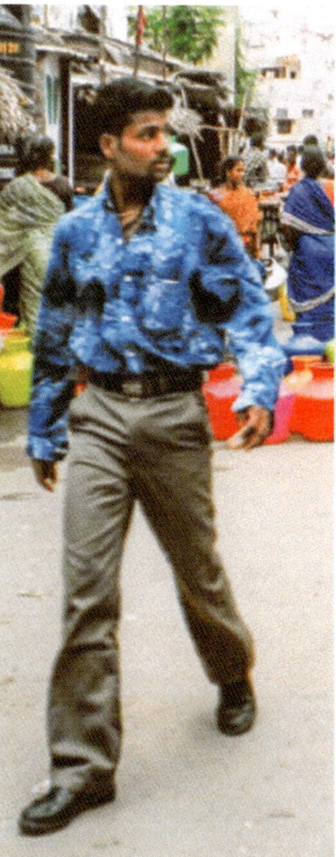

In Balance. The active leg is far back. Strong foot action propels it forward.

In Balance. The back foot contracts and the knee bends. The man at left has lifted his heel and his knee is about to bend. The man at right is pushing off with the tips of his toes, not with the ball of the foot.

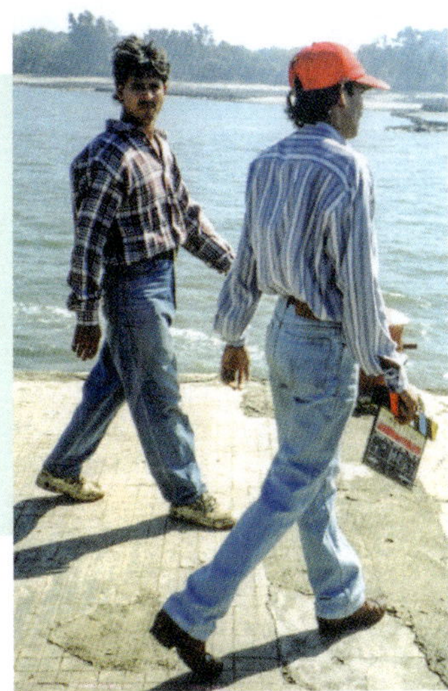

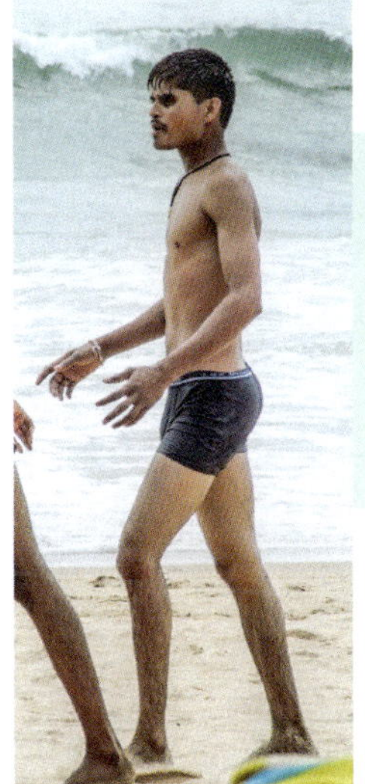

In Balance. All the action is in the back leg, foot, and buttocks. The back leg is straight and firm just before push-off.

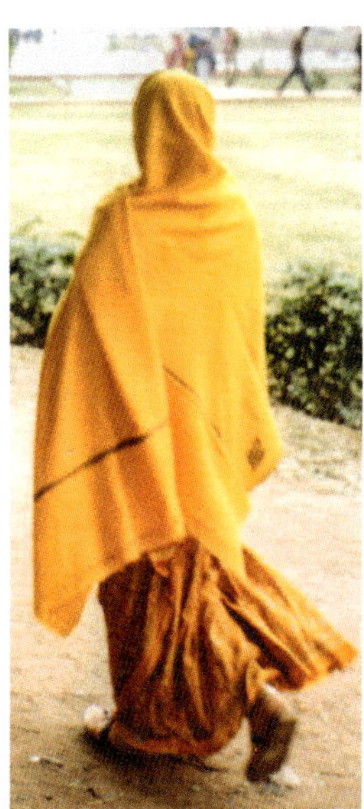

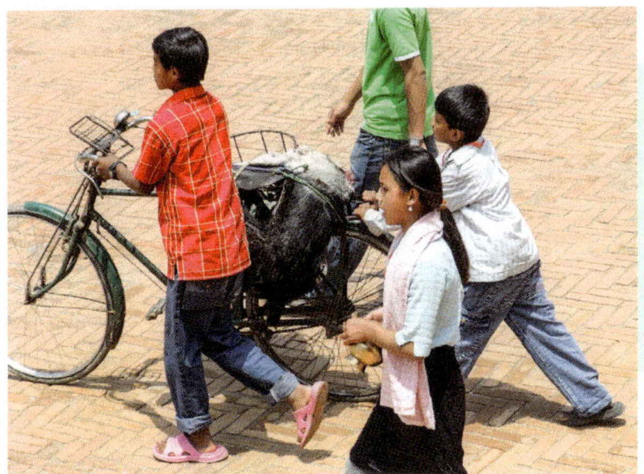

In Balance. After final push-off with the toes of the back foot, the knee bends and the foot lifts as if you are kicking up sand behind you.

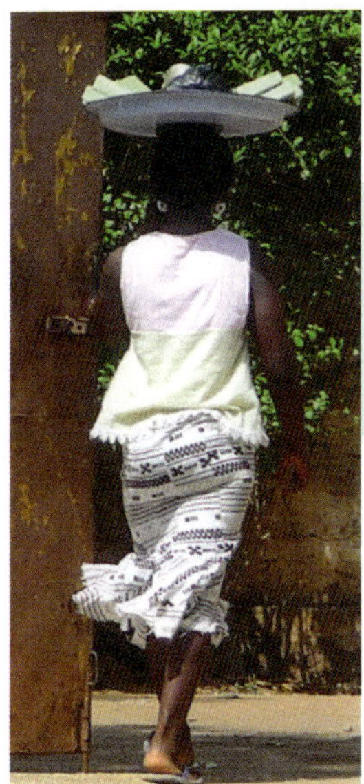

In Balance. The action in the buttocks is clearly visible in the rounding of the buttock muscles.

3. *Transferring your weight*

- Your left foot lands relatively flat, your heel touching the ground barely before your toes. Let the foot land with control and without making a sound.
- For a moment, when part of the weight is transferred, both feet touch the ground.
- A final push-off with the toes of the back foot puts the full weight on your front leg.
- When your front leg becomes weight-bearing, it straightens and moves back to begin a new step.

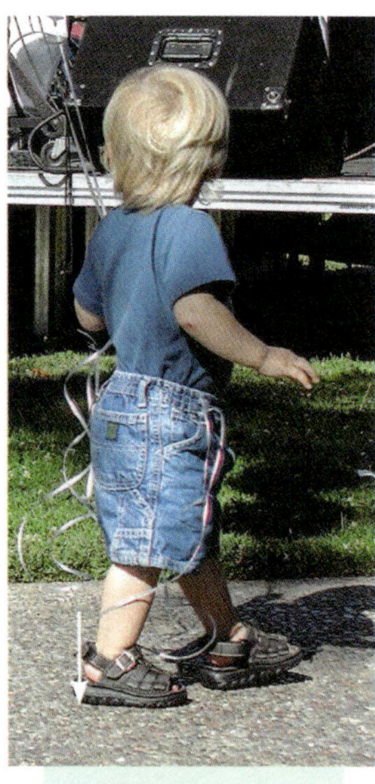

In Balance. For a moment, when part of the weight is transferred, both feet are on the ground.

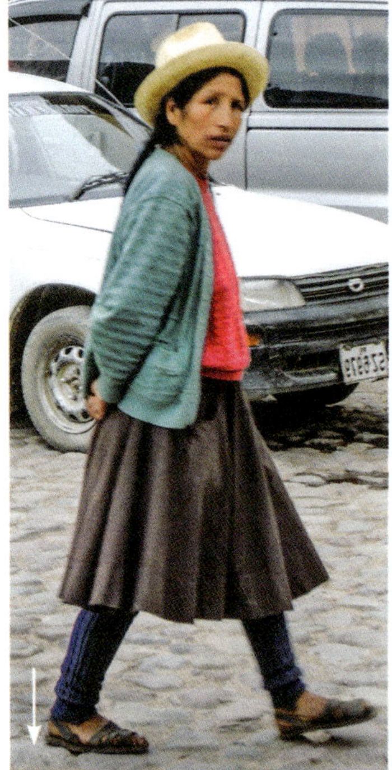

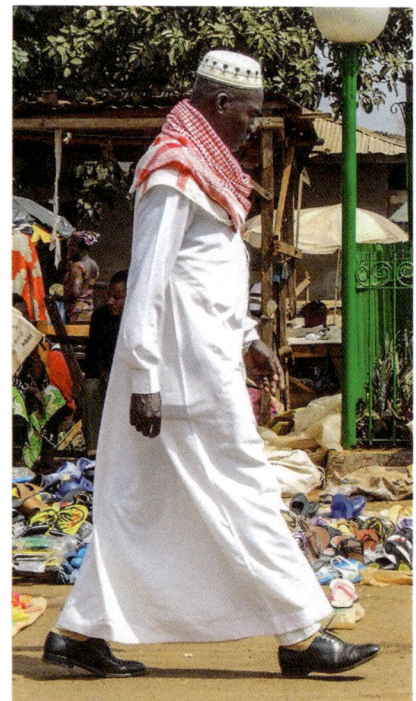

In Balance. The trunk stays upright and undisturbed. The whole back foot stays on the ground as the front leg moves forward. Your foot lands relatively flat, the heel touching the ground barely before the toes.

Walking: Putting It All Together

- Stand in Balance, weight in your heels.
- Transfer your weight to your right leg, weight in the heel.
- With a strong heel-to-toe contraction, lift your right heel and bend your knee. Push off.
- Simultaneously, let your left leg swing forward.
- While your back foot still touches the ground, your front leg lands with control.
- Your right leg passes through with a final push-off from the tips of the toes.
- Your left leg is now behind you, weight-bearing and straight.

CHECK AND FEEL

☑ *Do you walk with most weight on the balls of your feet, not in the heels?*

You are leaning back and your pelvis lifts in front; it is leading the way. The more you sit slightly when you walk, the more you will feel weight in your heels. Practice walking with your toes curled under while staying upright, and your pelvis will immediately rotate down between your legs. Feel the difference.

☑ *Do your knees hurt?*

Pain or strain in your knee may be due to locking your knee as you straighten your leg.

☑ *Does your low back hurt?*

Pain in the low back is often caused by arching your back and trying to stand straight. *Lengthen with the corselet* instead. Find a rhythm that keeps weight on your weight-bearing leg *as long as possible.* This works only when your pelvis stays rotated down in front, creating the sensation of walking as though you are slightly seated.

☑ *Do your buttocks stay soft?*

When the arches of your foot contract and your knee bends, your buttocks respond by contracting strongly—they feel firm. The contraction of your buttocks will happen naturally, but only if the pelvis stays down in front. Stay slightly seated.

TIPS FOR MORE PRACTICE

Swinging your free leg

- Bend your free leg at the knee and swing it back and forth a few times from your hip. Make this movement as smooth and light as possible.
- *Stay supported by your standing leg.* Resist leaning back or falling forward; stay centered.
- Switch sides and notice any difference in leg strength and ease of movement in the hip joint.

Pushing off

- Take a step back, equal weight in both legs. Contract your back foot, lift the heel, and bend the knee to feel the buttocks contract and become firm.

Reinforcing the forward-tilted position of the pelvis

- Walk a few steps on your heels with your toes lifted off the ground. Then repeat, but let your toes touch the ground. This helps you to feel weight in the heels.
- Walk without making the slightest sound.
- Walk backward. Notice the upright angle of your torso. Keep that angle and walk forward.
- Walk uphill. This will help you sense the feeling of walking slightly seated.

Putting it all together

- Try to copy the walking position in the photos, especially the strong leg and foot action and upright bearing without leaning back from your hips.

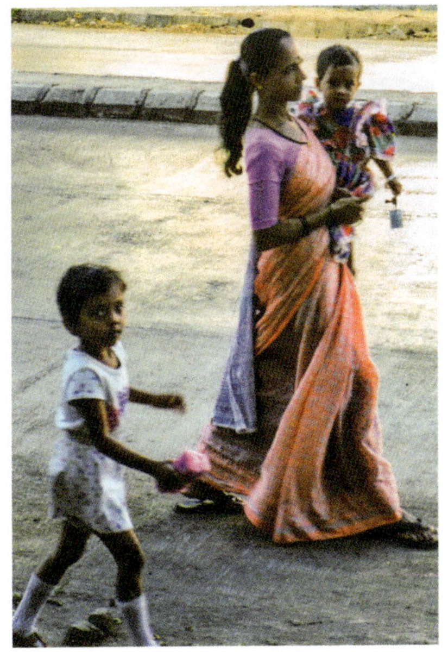

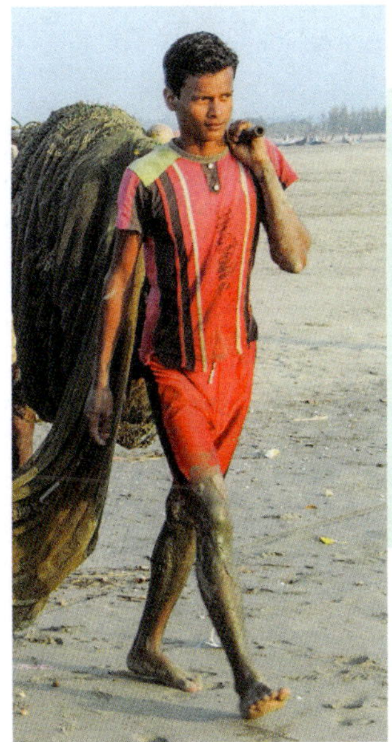

In Balance. (Left) While transferring weight there is a moment when both feet are on the ground. Notice the upright, regal bearing.

(Right) Before pushing off, the back leg is completely extended. Despite carrying a heavy weight on one shoulder, the shoulders and hips are horizontal and even.

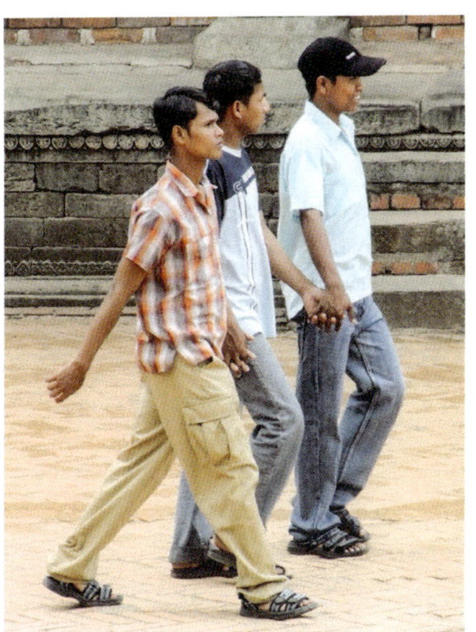

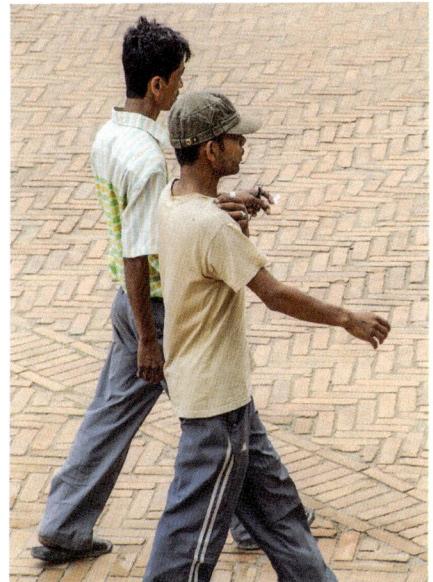

In Balance. Notice the strong leg action in all these men and how far the back leg extends behind them. As soon as the back heel lifts, the knee begins to bend.

LYING DOWN IN BALANCE

Detail and precision of the body lead to mastering the art of relaxation.

~ Noelle Perez-Christiaens[19]

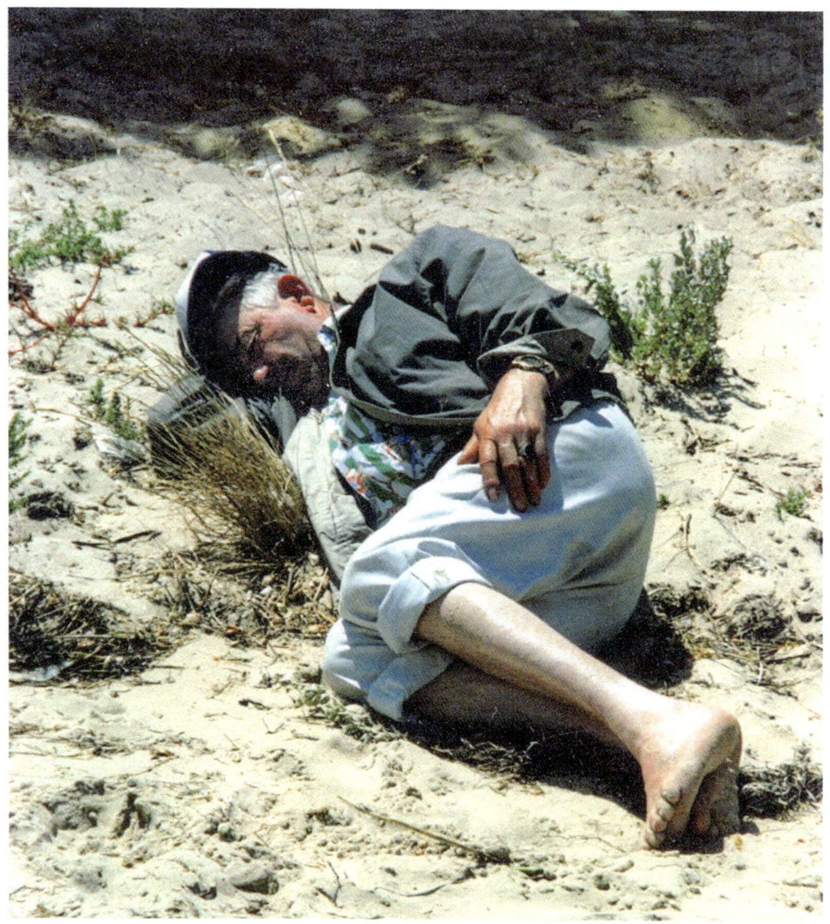

Resting on the beach, unfazed by the world around him.

Lying Down Comfortably Anywhere

In many countries it is not uncommon to see people lying down asleep on the beach, in a train station or airport, or even in the street. This is completely acceptable and practical in many cultures, especially in hot climates or when there is no other place to rest.

The sleepers have an uncanny way of relaxing, unfazed by the commotion all around. They seem able to fall asleep almost instantly—relaxation being the chief difference between people in and out of Balance.

The sleeping surface is usually hard—a stone floor, sandy beach, or wooden bench. But people almost always use some padding to elevate their head to keep it in alignment with the spine. If nothing can be found they use their bent arm as a pillow.

Their body posture is consistent: The pelvis is angled down in the front, as if sitting on a stool or chair. The back and neck are extended in a straight line, the chest is open, and the legs are bent with the knees raised no higher than the hips. They never lie in a fetal position.

Nöelle Perez-Christiaens observed in many instances that sleeping quarters in less industrialized countries may be more crowded than our own, but people's sleeping positions are not cramped.

What she learned from these relaxed sleepers can help us change habits that limit breathing, inhibit circulation, and interrupt sleep.

Lying on Your Side

As with sitting, placement of the pelvis is key. A fetal position inhibits circulation and continues the pattern of rounding the spine. A lengthened, straight spine opens up the chest and abdomen and enables deeper breathing.

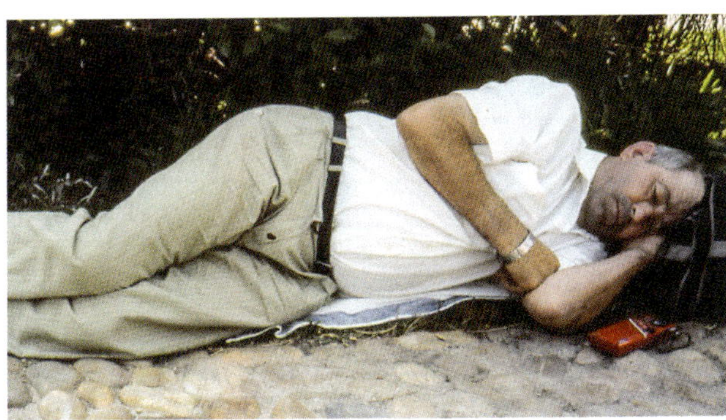

Necessity is often the mother of invention. On a hard surface this man has made himself comfortable with a thick pad or blanket under his rib cage and something to prop up his head.

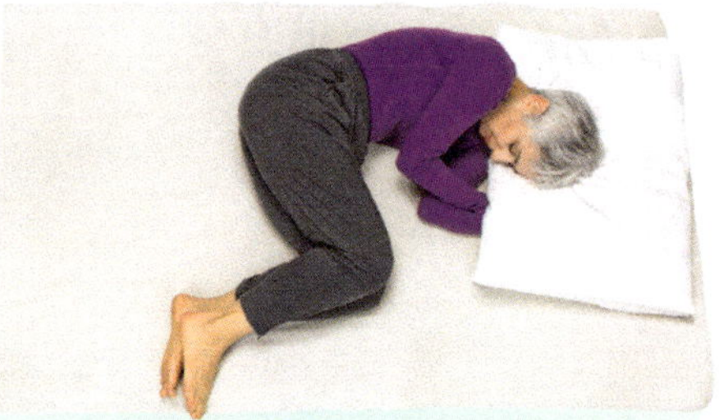

Out of Balance. The fetal position inhibits circulation and continues the pattern of rounding the spine.

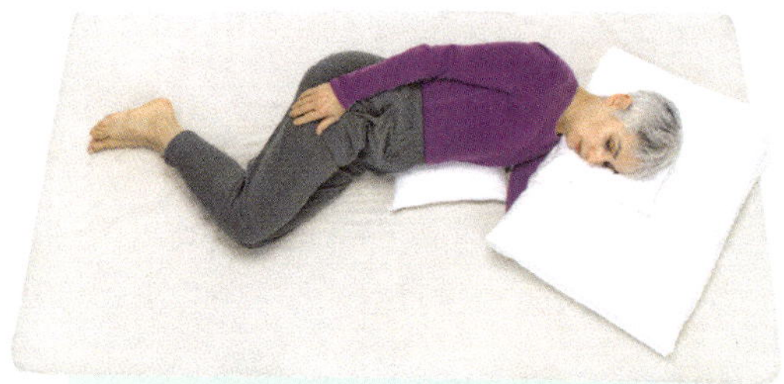

In Balance. The lengthened spine opens up the chest and abdomen and enables deeper breathing. Notice that the ankles are in line with the hips. Legs are usually together.

HOW TO PRACTICE

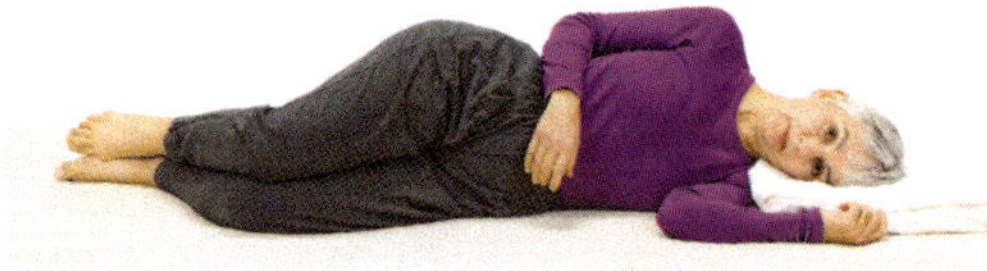

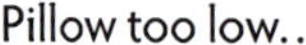

Pillow too low...

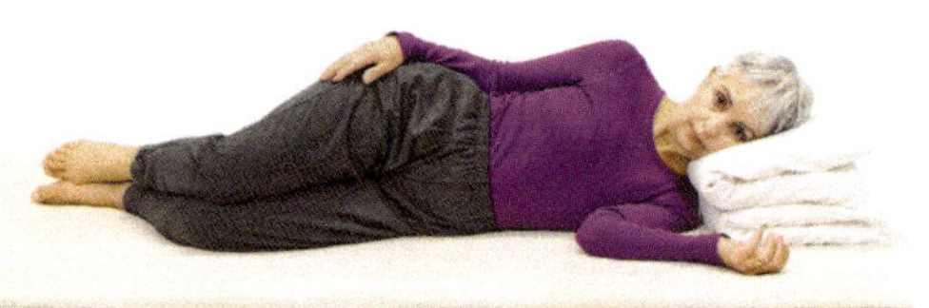

too high...

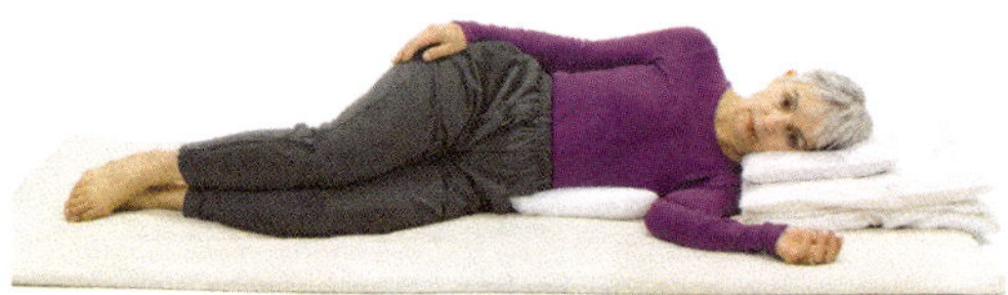

just right.

Figure 1

- Use a pillow (or more than one) that provides enough thickness to keep your neck extended in line with your spine and to fill the space between your ear and the floor or bed. Pull the pillow(s) tight against your shoulder so your neck is well supported *(figure 1).*

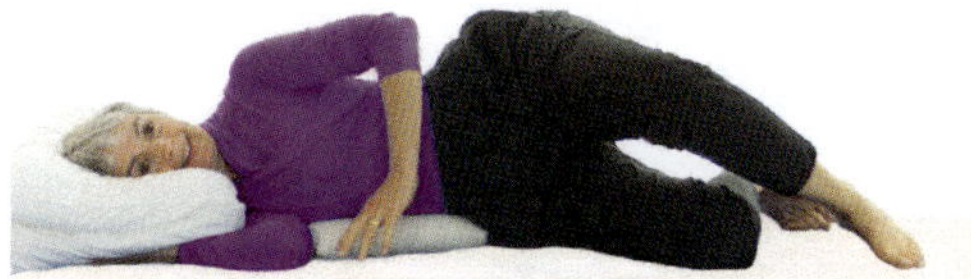

Figure 2

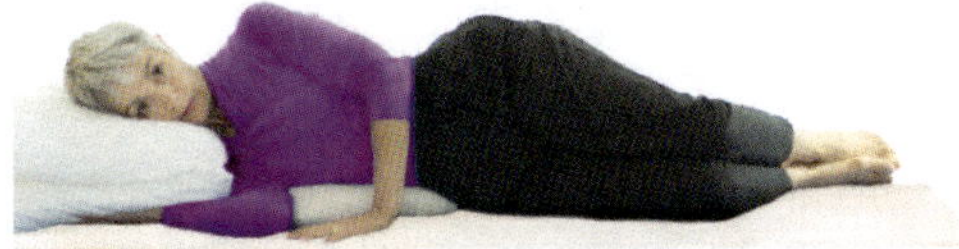

Figure 3

- Place your pelvis. Put your upper hand on the bed in front of you. Push down on your hand and feet to lift your pelvis and rotate the fig leaf down between your legs *(figure 2).*
- Then let go and relax your pelvis. Your legs should be at a diagonal angle with knees together, ankles directly below your hips *(figure 3).*

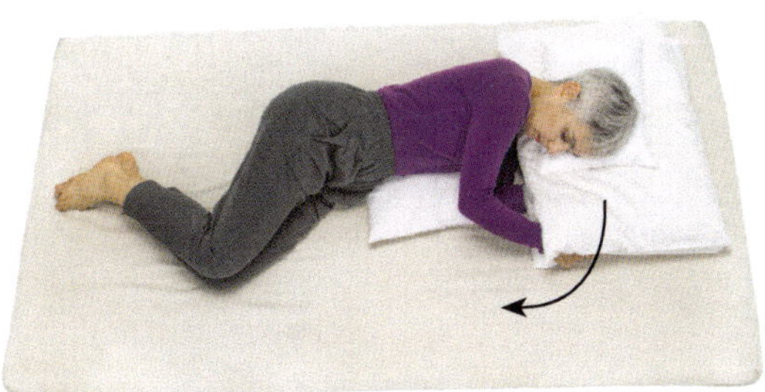

Figure 4

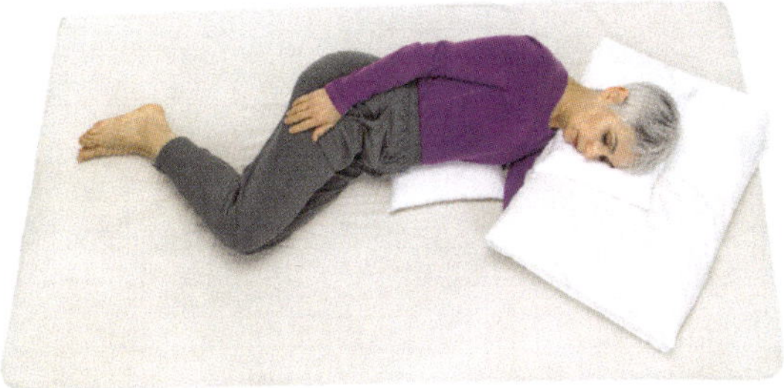

Figure 5

- Take hold of the bottom pillow corner next to your chin *(figure 4).* Pull the pillow corner down toward your chest, moving your head, pillow, and shoulders forward a little. This stretches out the lower back.
- Rest your arm on your upper side *(figure 5).*
- Feel length in the belly and back. Feel the breath in your back.

CHECK AND FEEL

☑ *Are your buttocks in front, rather than behind, your spine?*

Re-fig and take care not to lift your knees so high that they drag the pelvis into a tail-tucked (fetal) position. Never place your knees higher than if you were sitting in a chair.

☑ *Not comfortable yet?*

A small pillow between your knees may help to stabilize your hips.

Lying on Your Back

> *The best sign of a good Savasana (Corpse pose) is a feeling of deep peace and pure bliss. Savasana is a watchful surrendering of the ego. Forgetting oneself, one discovers oneself.*
>
> ~ Nöelle Perez-Christiaens[20]

To relax fully in a prone position we look for the same alignment as in all other positions: a forward pelvis, a natural arch, and a long extended spine and neck. To lengthen the spine and eliminate excess curving it is important to relax your chest and back. This is greatly helped by pillows under the head and edge of the shoulders, so that both are lifted forward enough to undo excess curving of the lumbar spine (low back) and neck. (See Using Pillows on page 103.)

HOW TO PRACTICE

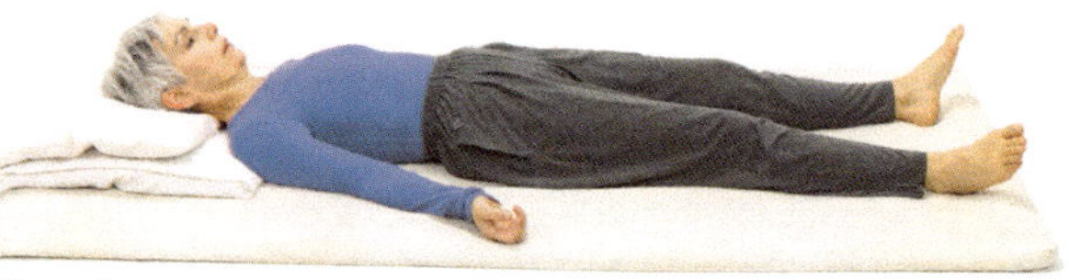

Figure 1

- Before you begin, set up two pillows or blankets, one a little lower than the other. The lower pillow supports the edge of your shoulders. Both pillows support your head *(figure 1).*

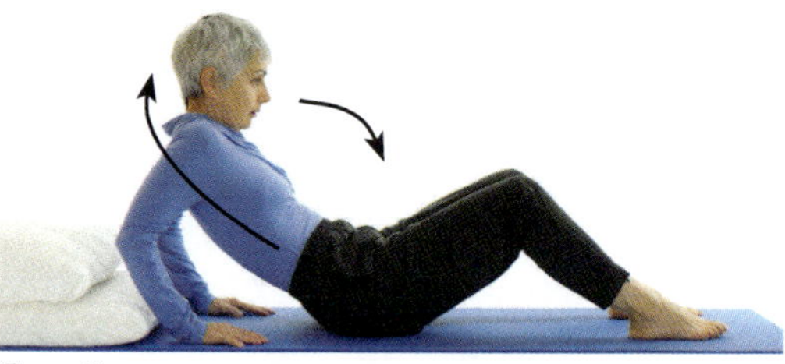

Figure 2

- To lie down, sit with bent knees, then fig (taking your pubic bone down between your legs) *(figure 2).*

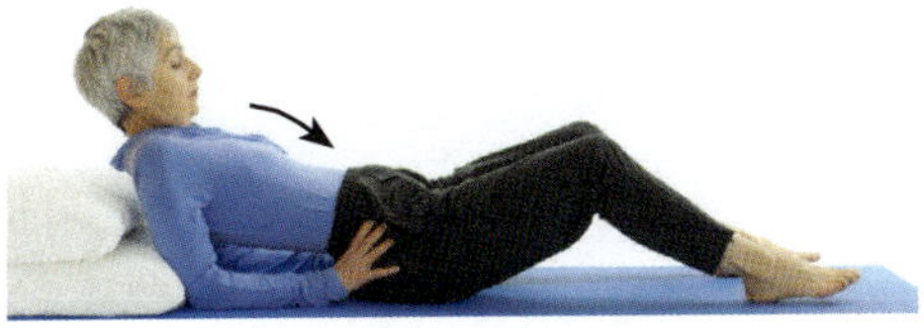

Figure 3

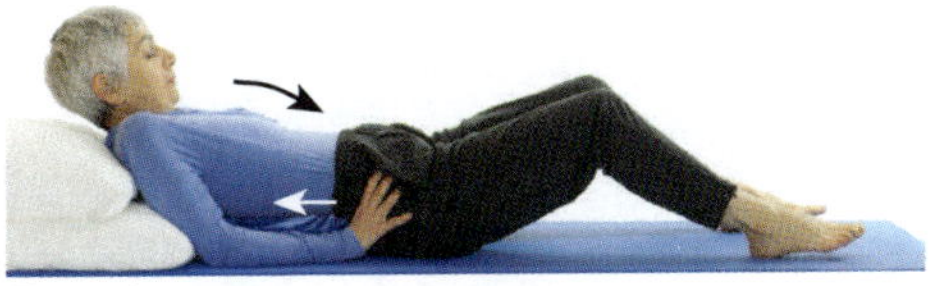

Figure 4

- Lean back on your elbows and fold down under your breasts *(figure 3)*. You will feel rounded. Hold this position while lowering yourself onto the bed, low back first, head last *(figure 4)*. Feel length in your low back.

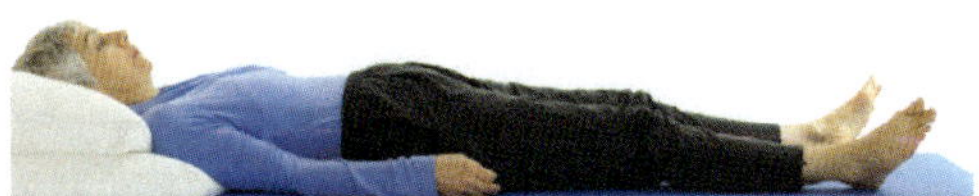

Figure 5

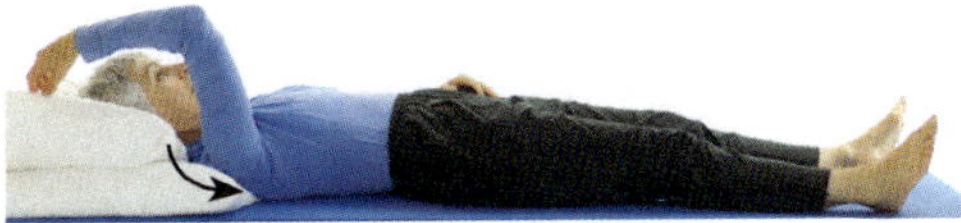

Figure 6

- Arrange the pillows so that your head is higher than your shoulders, and your forehead higher than your chin *(figure 5)*.
- Slide the base of your skull upward to lengthen your neck and angle your chin down.
- On each side: Lift one arm up to your ear and feel your shoulder blade flatten. Return the arm to your side *(figure 6)*.
- Relax everywhere and feel your breath as an up-and-down movement in your back.

CHECK AND FEEL

☑ *Is the breath in your back?*

If you feel no movement in your back when you breathe, experiment with the height of the pillows. More height will elevate your upper torso, flattening the arch in your spine. When the spine is extended your breath circulates freely in your chest, sides, and back with barely any movement in the belly. The diaphragm moves up and down rather than in and out, so that each breath massages your spine.

USING PILLOWS

The only way to lengthen the back is to shorten the front. We do this by lengthening the spine as we lie down and keeping it long with enough pillows so that the chest and the chin do not lift.

How do you know how high the pillows should be?

The test is your breath. If your chest expands freely and completely all the way to the top as you inhale, your spine is long and the chest cavity is free to expand. If instead your belly expands and there is little movement in your chest, you need more height to bring head and shoulders farther forward.

WHERE TO GO FROM HERE

When the student is ready, the teacher will appear.

The simplest, most effective way to use the guidelines in this book is to be present while going about your daily activities. Listen, interpret, and learn to respond to your body's messages of pain, fatigue, and tension. Know when to question and when to pull back or continue on. You choose, because you know best.

Think of Balance as the yoga of everyday life. With reflection, awareness, and attention you will find that even mundane activities like standing in line, sitting in a waiting room, or going for a walk become opportunities to observe, test, and explore.

Keep in mind that Balance is not a rigid, fixed posture. It is a point of reference. Gradually you will begin to feel taller, stronger, lighter, and better about how you look. Balance offers you a path toward maintaining your health, feeling vibrant and energetic, and aging gracefully and without pain. Balance introduces profound change. It is empowering!

Key Reminders

Jean Couch and her teachers at the Balance Center have developed short phrases to remind students of key actions to practice again and again. You've seen these throughout the book:

- *Hinge at the hips.* Whenever you bend, pivot from your hips and keep your back from rounding.
- *Fig* each time you sit down. Sit with your buttocks well underneath and behind you.
- *Ribs down.* If your back feels tight, your ribs are lifted.
- *Look at your ankles* when you stand, letting your legs move back. Feel weight in your heels. Straighten your knees but keep them soft.
- *Sit a little* when you stand or walk, keeping the pelvis relaxed downward in front.
- *Follow the line.* Think tall. Keep extending and lengthening the spine in all you do.

The following Golden Rules are helpful to keep in mind.

GOLDEN RULES

***Discover* tension and discomfort.**

Become aware of your habits, and tensions will begin to register. For instance, instead of fidgeting in a chair, begin to feel your discomfort (probably unnoticed before) and change how you sit. Instead of forcing yourself to sit through pain, understand when and why something hurts and what you must do to change a pain-inducing pattern.

***Undo* rather than do.**

We tend to strive for improvement through effort, asking, Which exercises can I do more of? Instead, focus on doing less with just the right amount of effort. When you discover a habit that saps your energy or causes pain, change it. You will find that undoing is more difficult than doing! Where you feel tightness, pain, or tension, relax there.

***Use the axis* as a guide.**

Visualize the axis of gravity by lifting up along a center line toward an imaginary weight on your head. This simple reminder helps to correct habits of asymmetrical movement, such as slouching or leaning to one side.

Doing Yoga and Working with a Teacher

You might want to explore beginning yoga poses to keep yourself limber, always keeping the guidelines for Balance in mind. If you already practice yoga, you will need to adapt your poses to the guidelines for Balance. A certified Balance teacher can give you feedback that will help you progress and keep you safe. Most Balance teachers are also students and teachers of yoga.

If possible, find a teacher to take you through the basics presented in this book. See Teacher Resources below.

TEACHER RESOURCES

Balance Center
560 Oxford Avenue
Palo Alto, California 94306
Phone: 650.856.2000
www.BalanceCenter.com

The Balance Center maintains a close relationship with the Aplomb Institute (ISA) in Paris (www.isaplomb.org). What the Balance Center teaches is based on Nöelle Perez-Christiaens' research. Nöelle's work is always evolving and she continues to share new insights. Balance teachers stay current by attending Nöelle's classes in Paris and annual workshops taught at the Balance Center by her senior teachers.

The Balance Center offers classes in the Foundations of Balance, Continuing Balance, Yoga in Balance, and Teacher Training. The Center also offers private lessons and special workshops at locations throughout the U.S.

Contact the Balance Center to find a teacher in your area.

Thea Sawyer
Phone: 408.489.9436
www.LiveInBalance.com

Thea Sawyer teaches Balance, Yoga in Balance, and Yoga for People with MS. She teaches in her private studio in San Jose, California, at the Balance Center, and at other Silicon Valley locations.

AFTERWORD

We at the Balance Center are so happy to welcome Thea Sawyer's book of Aplomb and Balance guidelines. We have needed this book ever since we had our first students in 1992. It is clear and concise, with pictures that inspire and instruct.

Discovering Balance was a huge relief for me. I had spent 20 years studying, teaching, and writing about Iyengar yoga. In 1979, a seminal year, I studied in Pune, India with B. K. S. Iyengar and my book, *Runner's World Yoga Book,* was published. Yet throughout this time, no matter what I practiced and taught, my posture was atrocious (swaybacked in the low spine, a stiff hump in my upper back, and a dowager's hump at the base of my neck). I also suffered from recurring bouts of painful sciatica. It puzzled me that yoga had no healing effect on these symptoms, and they were getting worse.

I know now, from the profound teachings of Nöelle Perez-Christiaens, that yoga was not the problem. It was the way I was doing yoga. Balance has solved the problem.

When Balance magically came into my life, I perceived almost instantly that it would address the condition of my spine like no other system. Right away I looked better and found that a few shifts in the position of my bones lessened the curve in my spine. When something hurt, I would say to myself, What if I tried shifting my position in this new way? Invariably I felt better.

When I started teaching even the simplest of Balance guidelines, students reported how much better they felt. I soon became fervent about Balance.

You too can get rid of long term, chronic aches and pains. Almost simultaneously you will begin to regain your natural strength. The more you do the better you will feel. Over time, the rewards of Balance become more profound. You experience yourself as lighter, and everything you do becomes easier.

I can't encourage you enough. The rewards are immense. Begin to explore these guidelines and enjoy yourself. This book is for you.

Jean Couch, Director
Balance Center
Palo Alto, California
www.BalanceCenter.com

NOTES

1. Institut Supérieur d'Aplomb, www.isaplomb.org.
2. Nöelle Perez-Christiaens, *Sparks of Divinity,* 215.
3. Nöelle obtained a PhD at the Ecole des Hautes Etudes en Sciences Sociales in Paris, Department of Social Anthropology and Ethnology.
4. Perez-Christiaens, *Sparks of Divinity,* 218.
5. Genevieve Brady, *The Human Form Divine,* 45.
6. Maud Smith Williams, *Growing Straight,* 10. A 1930 book about "a new system of physical education as practiced by North American Indians."
7. Brady, *The Human Form Divine,* 38.
8. Doris Lessing, *African Laughter.* In this memoir, British-born Lessing recalls her childhood in former Rhodesia, now Zimbabwe. She recounts her visits in the 1980s and '90s after being exiled for 25 years.
9. Perez-Christiaens, *Etre d'Aplomb,* 9.
10. Williams, *Growing Straight,* 42.
11. H. Rouviere and A. Delmas, *Anatomie Humaine, Tome 2.*
12. L. Testut, *Traite d'Anatomie Humaine.*
13. Quoted by Perez-Christiaens, *Sparks of Divinity,* 92.
14. Perez-Christiaens, *Etre d'Aplomb,* 19.
15. Ibid., 109.
16. Williams, *Growing Straight,* 48.
17. Lessing, *African Laughter.*
18. Harriet Doerr, *Consider This, Señora.*
19. Perez-Christiaens, *Sparks of Divinity,* 96.
20. Ibid., 104.

GLOSSARY

alignment The distribution of weight along a central line. With proper alignment this median line divides the torso into symmetrical halves.

Aplomb From the French, meaning "plumb"; adhering to a plumb line. Used by Nöelle Perez-Christiaens to describe a natural uprightness in line with gravity, as measured by a plumb line. Natural means *being* upright, rather than *holding* oneself upright.

axis of gravity The direction of up; the universal plumb line. The line of gravity is an imaginary vertical line that extends upward and downward from an object's center of gravity. When a person is standing in Balance, seen in profile, the line of gravity can be considered as a plumb line that passes through the middle of the head to the heels via the midhip (trochanter) and the natural arch (low lumbar area) of the spine.

Balance The optimal alignment of our bones in space and an optimal distribution of weight. Synonymous with Aplomb.

cervical spine The first seven vertebrae of the spine, forming the neck.

corselet French for a small corset; refers to the muscles that support the trunk and the spine like an inner corset. These are the abdominal muscles that work in harmony with the muscles of the spine. To engage the corselet is to activate the abdominal muscles to lift and lengthen the spine and stabilize the trunk.

extended spine A lengthened spine with an even groove down the center of the back from the upper shoulders to the sacrum and relaxed muscles on either side.

fig; figging The action of moving the pubic bone (the "fig leaf") down and back between the legs so the weight is in the front of the pelvis.

follow the line A reminder to think tall, to extend and lengthen the spine along its axis in all you do. See **axis of gravity.**

forward-rotated pelvis A pelvis that slopes forward and down. Visualize a belt line that angles down toward the front.

hip socket The joint where the trunk hinges on the legs to facilitate bending forward. To locate the hip socket, touch the crease where your leg meets your trunk; in the center is your hip socket.

in Balance Healthy posture with the following characteristics: a forward-rotated pelvis, a long spine with an evenly formed groove down its center, the front ribs relaxed down toward the spine, the shoulders extending straight out to the sides, a downward angled chin, and a long neck. In Balance there is no friction, no resistance to gravity. There is only ease.

look at your ankles A reminder to rotate the pelvis forward and down until you are standing with weight in the heels. You do this by letting the tops of your legs move back far enough to see your ankles.

lumbar spine The five vertebrae that form the third section of the spine, around the waist. It is the place where modern spines tend to have an overly long, "false" curve, resulting in a hollow back. The low lumbar spine is the most frequently injured part of the back.

natural arch The small curvature at the base of the lumbar spine, where the spine and sacrum meet. The natural arch encompasses vertebrae S1, L5, and L4. Nöelle Perez-Christiaens found this to be the "true" lumbar curve (not encompassing all five lumbar vertebrae).

pelvis The pelvis forms the base of the trunk and is shaped like a bowl, formed by the pubic bone in front, the hip bones at the sides, and the sacrum in the back. The position of the pelvis is critical for alignment of the spine.

ribs down Relaxing the chest by settling the ribs downward toward the spine.

sacrum The five fused vertebrae at the tail end of the spine. Together they form a triangular bone and the back side of the pelvis.

sit a little A reminder to let the pelvis relax downward in front when you are standing or walking, so that you feel as if you are slightly seated.

sitting bones *(ischial tuberosities)* Two curved bones that extend from the base of the pelvis, forming its lower end. Feel them underneath when sitting upright, especially when rocking side to side or front to back.

thoracic spine The twelve vertebrae that form the second section of the spine, from the base of the neck to the midback.

BIBLIOGRAPHY

Brady, Genevieve. *The Human Form Divine.* New York, 1920.

Calais-Germain, Blandine. *Anatomy of Movement.* Seattle: Eastland Press, 1993.

Doerr, Harriet. *Consider This, Señora.* New York: Harcourt Brace & Company, 1993.

Lessing, Doris. *African Laughter.* New York: HarperCollins, 1992.

Perez-Christiaens, Nöelle. *Etincelles de Divinite.* Paris: Institut Supérieur d'Aplomb, 1976.

——. *Etre d'Aplomb.* Paris: Institut Supérieur d'Aplomb, 1983.

——. *Sparks of Divinity.* Berkeley, CA: Rodmell Press, 2012.

——. *Thus Spake B.K.S. Iyengar.* Paris: Institut de Yoga B.K.S. Iyengar, 1979.

Rolf, Ida P. *Rolfing.* Rochester, VT: Healing Arts Press, 1989.

Rouviere, H., and A. Delmas. *Anatomie Humaine, Tome 2.* Paris: Masson, 1992.

Testut, L. *Traité d'Anatomie Humaine.* Paris: Octave Doin et Fils, 1911.

Williams, Maud Smith. *Growing Straight.* New York: A.S. Barnes and Company, 1930.

INDEX

ABOUT THE AUTHOR

Thea Sawyer is a Certified Balance Instructor (1992), a certified Aplomb Instructor (1997), and a California-certified yoga teacher (2002). Born and raised in Holland, she has lived in New York, San Francisco, Buenos Aires, Paris, and San Jose, California. Her empirical studies of healthy posture have taken her to Mexico, Argentina, India, Portugal, France, and The Netherlands.

Before discovering Balance, Thea lived with chronic back pain, scoliosis, and lumbar disk damage that limited her activities and sapped her energy. Especially debilitating symptoms during her years as a computer programmer led her to begin studying Balance in 1991. In 1996 she moved to Paris to study with Nöelle Perez-Christiaens at the Aplomb Institute. She also completed an anthropology research project at the University of Paris and received a diploma from the Ecole des Hautes Etudes en Sciences Sociales (1997).

Thea has studied therapeutic yoga at the Mandiram (therapeutic yoga center) of TKV Desikachar in India and with Kate Holcombe in San Francisco.

Today Thea's back pains are gone, she feels more fit than ever, and the healing powers of Aplomb and Balance have made her a passionate practitioner of these techniques. She loves to share her knowledge of pain-free posture and how to maintain energy and ease of movement at any age.

Thea Sawyer teaches Balance, Yoga in Balance, and Yoga for People with MS in her private studio in San Jose, California, at the Balance Center, and at other Silicon Valley locations. This is her first book.

Made in the USA
Charleston, SC
01 April 2014